Optimal Prescription Health

THE REAL TRUTH
about balancing your prescription with complementary medicines

HOW A GOOD PHARMACIST
CAN SAVE YOUR LIFE

MARTIN HARRIS
Leading Pharmacist and
Nutrition Medicine Expert

What Others Are Saying...

Before I came for treatment with Martin I was bloated, lethargic, had lots of phlegm and couldn't sleep without sleeping pills. Now after some treatments I have much less bloating. I have lots more energy and a clear chest. I am now sleeping without sleeping pills – such a relief! I have referred my friends to Martin.

—Jan Turley

On another note, the supplements that you have given me are already making an enormous difference! I have been following the guidelines for slowly introducing one at a time, but even just the few days on the the Pro-Biotic and the Gut Ease have made such a remarkable difference. I no longer bloat and swell up after every meal, and digestion as a whole is just so much more comfortable, without the cramping and gas etc. I appeared to just be getting worse and worse before seeing you, and this is the first time in months that I have been free of digestion problems! So, already I am so grateful to be relieved of these symptoms!

—Lauryn Buchanan

"Thanks very much for the video information you have on the TV monitor in the store. Even after only one week on the magnesium powder, I felt the benefits. I rested better at night and found that I didn't have that 'already tired' feeling when I get up every morning. After a month on the magnesium powder, I don't get any of those nightly leg cramps. Thank you for your advice."

—Marley Bearden

Martin Harris

BPharm, RegPharmNZ, MBA (Distinction), AACNEM, PGCert Nutrition Medicine (Distinction).

Martin Harris, pharmacist, nutrition medicine expert, and author, is passionate and committed to helping people achieve optimal health and wellness through safe and proven nutrition medicine strategies.

Martin has experience in a wide variety of health fields, starting his career in a community pharmacy setting. He then spent time as the Editor of an international drug information review journal, has written many evaluations of new and existing medicines, and worked in marketing and senior management teams within the pharmaceutical industry. To round out his perspective on the health industry, Martin has also spent five years advising the New Zealand Government on pharmaceutical management.

His quest for the answers to health and vitality were inspired by his family's tragic health story. Watching helplessly as conventional medicine failed to provide solutions to his father's and his wife's major health crises was one of the hardest things he has had to face. This inspired Martin to retrain under the leading nutrition medicine experts in Australasia, and set up his own nutrition medicine clinic.

Now Martin sees the same illness cycle that plagued his family mirrored in many of his patients in his pharmacy and nutrition medicine clinic. But the exciting part is that the formal learning and practical experience that Martin has acquired over more than 20 years is providing outstanding solutions to help these people.

Now Martin wants to raise the awareness of pitfalls of a "blinkered" approach to health to a wider audience and has written this book to share this knowledge with you.

Lifestyle Practitioner Academy
Private Practice Marketing Pty Ltd
PO Box 1131
Byron Bay NSW 2481

For information regarding Optimal Prescription Health
please contact Martin Harris +64 9-833-7239
or e-mail *help@masseyamcal.co.nz*

ISBN-13: 978-1463527457
ISBN-10: 1463527454

Acknowledgements

There are three people that I will single out to acknowledge for their contribution to this book. If any of these people were not in my life, I do not think I would have written this book.

To my wife, Christine, for the support and belief in me and what I am trying to achieve, especially when it must have seemed a little "left field" on occassions.

To Adam Gibson for helping me to realize that I have a responsibility to share my knowledge with the world through writing this book.

To Professor Mel Sydney-Smith for sharing his extensive knowledge of health that he has acquired from his lifetime of performing health miracles for patients.

There are many other people that have also helped me and I am grateful for their input into my life.

Special Bonus Offer

Nutricheck Health Analysis

For you and a loved one

Plus a 20 minute personal health consultation

(either face-to-face or via Skype or Phone)

(Valued at $280)

*A Nutricheck Health Analysis is an important step
in your journey to wellness.*

What the Nutricheck Health Analysis will do for you:

- You will discover how likely it is that your health condition is actually caused by a deficiency of one or more nutrients.
- You will discover what nutrients your body is crying out for.
- Your Nutricheck report will reveal if your prescription drugs have caused low levels of essential nutrients.
- You will receive your own personalized plan to assist you to achieve Optimal Health.

As a bonus gift for investing in this book, you can claim your FREE GIFT of a Nutricheck Health Analysis.

To claim your Nutricheck Health Analysis please register at:
www.OptimalPrescriptionHealth.co.nz

This offer is open to all acquirers of Optimal Prescription Health, The Real Truth About Balancing Your Prescription With Complementary Medicines, How A Good Pharmacist Can Save Your Life, by Martin Harris. Original proof of purchase is required. This offer is limited to the Nutricheck Health Analysis and a 20 minute consultation only (in person, or remotely by Phone or Skype), and your appointment will be subject to availability of appointments. The appointments must be completed by **1 December 2012**. The value of this Nutricheck Health Analysis for you and a loved one is $280 as of April 2011. While book purchasers will be responsible for the travel, meals, accommodation and other expenses, the Nutricheck Health Analysis is complimentary. In undertaking a Nutricheck Health Analysis you are under no obligation whatsoever to Martin Harris, his pharmacy or his clinic.

Contents

Contents

Preface

I'm Ashamed Of Myself!

Let me tell you a bit of my story of how I became what I am today; a pharmacist, nutrition medicine practitioner, optimal prescription health advisor, speaker and author.

My story will explain what has driven me to draw a line in the sand and scream out "ENOUGH!" Why I am ashamed to be a part of the health system that fails so many people. How extreme frustration has driven me to seek real answers to the health crisis that we are facing. My story will also reveal why I have taken action and chosen better health for my family and my patients.

Now I am on a crusade to bring the vital health information that I have discovered to as many people as possible. I feel it is my duty to share this information, which is why I have written this book. I feel a duty to help people understand for themselves what is causing their ill health and what they can do to treat these causes and help themselves. I feel responsible for making sure no-one suffers unnecessarily from the side effects of prescription medicines that could have been avoided. I also want to make sure that no-one misses out on a safe and effective treatment just because they weren't aware of it—at least not on my watch!

You may have guessed by now that I am extremely passionate about health. I focus this passion on helping people at both ends of the health spectrum. First, in my clinic I specialize in treating patients with very complex health conditions get better. Secondly, in my pharmacy I like to educate people about how they can achieve optimal health from their prescriptions as well as how to avoid complex health conditions. I am not aware of any other pharmacists doing this work, so that makes me a little unusual (probably in more ways than one!). The following sections describe how I became what I am today.

A Wide-Eyed Student Chooses His Career

I started my career as a pharmacist thinking I would be able to contribute to the health of people in my community. Before I chose pharmacy as a profession I thought that knowing how the body works, how medicines work and how medications and the body interact would be awesome. And now 25 years down the track I can tell you that the knowledge I have obtained is awesome. The more I learn, the more I can help people including my family. But there is more to it than I even imagined back in my youth.

The Harsh Realities Of The Workplace

After I finished my pharmacy degree, I went to work in a community pharmacy where I soon found the reality of the pharmacy workplace was a bit different to my rosy picture. Things were done at such a fast pace that I did not have time to think about the medicines I was dispensing or the people who were going to receive them. Admittedly, this was back in the 1980s, when the practice of pharmacy had yet to become more patient-centered.

I actually felt that during my first year working as a pharmacist I had forgotten a lot of what I had learned at University. You know what they say "use it or lose it." In fact, I started to wonder if I had actually learned it in the first place.

A Change Of Tack

So I decided to change tack and went to work for a company that specialized in producing drug information. This was great in that I started to relearn everything about pharmacology and how drugs affect the body as well as how the body affects drugs. In fact, I was even researching data on drugs that hadn't even been released yet.

It was great work for my development and confidence, since I was working with some of the best health experts throughout the world. But I missed the contact with real patients; patients with faces and personalities rather than just cohorts in a study.

Back To My Roots

So I headed back to community pharmacy. I was a little surprised when I went back to pharmacy as to how little had changed in terms of the health solutions available in the shop. There were the same old pain killers and cough medicines and nose sprays that I knew didn't work that well even 10 years earlier. I started to think that there must be some better solutions to people's health problems.

The other thing I noticed was the vitamin section. People started to ask me for my advice on vitamins and I had to confess that I didn't have much knowledge about them at all. We had not learned much about natural health, vitamins, nutrition or diet at Pharmacy School.

Back To School

I am not a person who likes to bluff my way through life without knowing the answers. So I thought I would learn all there was to know about natural health. I attended a few seminars, which whet my appetite for learning in this area. But I wanted to know everything "now." So I did some investigation and found the best natural health education course available. It was an intensive 5-day course in Australia run by a group of trail-blazing doctors.

Spending several thousand dollars and a week away from

home when you have a young family is not easy. But my wife (and my bank manager) was very understanding and supportive, so away I went to learn everything there was to know about natural health.

I Learned There Was More To Learn

The course that I did was the Australasian College of Nutritional and Environmental Medicine (ACNEM) primary course. It was a fantastic course and I learned heaps. In fact, when I got home at midnight, I talked excitedly to my wife in bed for several hours about many of the things that I had learned. I think I nearly burned her ears with my excitement.

One of the most important lessons that I learned at the ACNEM Primary Course was how much more there was to know. So I kept going to seminars and I eventually attended a seminar by one of the world's best nutrition medicine specialists, Professor Mel Sydney-Smith. He inspired me with stories of the power of nutrition medicine and his detailed and methodical approach to assessing patients. In fact, I was so inspired that I enrolled in a degree that he was teaching called the Master of Nutrition Medicine degree that was being run in conjunction with RMIT University.

The Nutrition Medicine Clinic Is Born

I was about a third of my way through the Master of Nutrition Medicine programme when it dawned on me that there was no use learning all this fantastic material if I wasn't going to use it to its full potential. So as well as helping my friends and family with my new knowledge, I cleared out the mezzanine floor of the pharmacy that had been used for storage. We refitted it as The Nutrition Medicine Clinic.

Much of my time is now taken up seeing patients with very serious health concerns in the clinic. I did start my clinic practice seeing patients from the pharmacy who wanted some better answers. However, as things have progressed I now get most of my patients referred to me from doctors. It is a great team approach working with open-minded doctors to get the patient feeling well. My patients are quite challenging cases that the doctors haven't got the time to investigate and treat as thoroughly as they would like. For example, setting up a new diet for a patient can take hours in itself. My clinic now employs two naturopaths and medical herbalists and one massage therapist in addition to me.

The Future

Right now I'm enjoying the challenges of my clinical practice as well as helping people in the pharmacy. Running both the clinic and the pharmacy is not without its stresses, but the success stories from my patients make it worthwhile. Going forward, I would like to help people avoid getting chronically ill by educating them about their health while they are still healthy. Or at least educate them about their health when they are only mildly ill. I've found people who are totally healthy often think they are bullet-proof and don't make good listeners! They are a challenge for another day.

This Book

This book marks the start of my new venture into educating people about their health. In this book I am open about the short comings of the health system and the health industry as a whole. I do not do this to be sensational, or to be critical of any individual people. Rather I feel a responsibility to let people know that the current health model might not provide the best health outcomes. I would rather offend some people than get to the end of my life and realize I didn't help all the people that I could have. I am proposing a new way of looking at health that utilizes the best of all worlds. I hope by reading this book, you or someone you love might stay well, or if they are already ill, then get better, sooner.

—Martin Harris

P.S. I encourage you to register for my free newsletter to help you to keep up-to-date with what is new in the world of health. Go to www.OptimalPrescriptionHealth.co.nz to register.

Revealing The Truth:
Why Our Health System Is Failing Real People

Medicine Helps But Can Also Cause Many Problems

There is a lot of research on the potential dangers of prescription medicines. The statistics are frightening. In one study published in the prestigious British Medical Journal, over 6% of all hospital admissions were directly related to prescription medicines. That means that there would be hundreds of people a day in New Zealand and Australia who end up in hospital because of problems with their prescription medicine.

There has been a lot of research on hospitalizations, since it is easy to track these patients. However, there is very little research on how many people just feel lousy while taking prescription medicines. In other words, we know there are lots of people that have serious adverse reactions to prescription medicines, but we don't know how many people just feel lousy. I would estimate from my work with tens of thousands of patients in my pharmacy and in my clinic over more than 20 years, that there are lots of people in this category who feel less than 100% well.

Similarly, there is very little information on how many people end up with a worse condition because of their prescription medicine. But in my pharmacy, I regularly see patients who are falling through the cracks of our conventional health system. These are people that start with a medical problem and receive medicine that helps alleviate the symptoms, but does not address the underlying causes of their ill health, or worse still is making their underlying health condition worse.

Then there is a third category of people that would benefit from reading this book. These are people that do not know that diet, lifestyle and nutrition can be even more effective than many prescription medicines ... and a lot safer too! Many people do understand there are effective complements or alternatives to taking a prescription medicine, but they don't know how to get quality unbiased information. Preventing this epidemic of medicine-induced ill health, and ensuring people can achieve optimal health is the goal of my book.

The Most Common Medicines Are The Worst Culprits

The most common medications that pharmacies dispense can actually make the underlying condition for which they are used worse. I know that this sounds incredible, like it's out of some scary conspiracy movie. I talk about some of these key medicines in detail in later chapters. But the key message I want you to understand at this stage, is that just because everyone else you know is on the same medicines as you, this doesn't mean that those medicines are the right ones for you. In fact, they could be doing you harm.

Now I am conscious of the fact that I might be creating a lot of worry for people taking prescription medicines. I certainly do not want you to stop taking any of your prescription medicines without first talking to your doctor and pharmacist. Not all prescription medicines are bad. Some do a great job with very few side effects.

My plea to you is to read through my book and get informed about the potential risks of prescription medicines and what you can do to lessen those risks. This book is not intended as a complete DIY guide to optimal prescription health, but rather to alert you to what is possible. I recommend you seek qualified advice before changing your medications or starting any nutrition supplements.

A Common Way That Medicines Cause Problems

At pharmacy school we studied pharmacology, which was broken down into two main areas:

1. How the body affects the drug.
2. How the drug affects the body.

One of the big holes in our training was the impact that drugs can have on the level of nutrients in the body. This is significant because it is often these very nutrients, including vitamins and minerals, that are needed to make the body work. After all, the name vitamin means vital for life. So by depleting key nutrients, some medications can actually make the underlying disease condition worse, or even trigger another disease process.

Is This An Industry Beat-Up? Should We Sack All The Doctors And Pharmacists?

My reasons for writing this book are not to cast blame on individuals in any profession, whether that is doctors, pharmacists, or natural health practitioners. My intention in this book is to highlight a significant health problem to make people aware of it. Like a lot of problems, once we bring it out in the open and start to talk about it, then the solutions become apparent. So my rationale is actually to help people understand how to get the best from their prescription medicine.

How The Drive For Efficiency Has Backfired

The problem is not because of bad prescription writing by doctors or sloppy dispensing by pharmacists. The problem lies with "the system." You see doctors and pharmacists are encouraged to work efficiently in a health system that has scarce resources. This means that doctors must see patients in their allotted 6 to 10 minute time slots. How crazy is that? Six minutes is not enough time to truly figure out what is wrong with a patient! Let alone make a plan of how to identify the underlying causes of illness and what to do about them.

The irony of this situation is that some patients do not respond well to our efficient health system. These are the patients who go from doctor to doctor, specialist to specialist. They have almost every laboratory test imaginable. And they end up costing the government much more than it would have cost to have taken the time and trouble to understand their condition early on.

My Pharmacy Patients Gang Up On Me

The efficiency race is even worse for a pharmacist. To be financially viable, a pharmacist needs to be dispensing a prescription medicine every four minutes. As a pharmacist, I can tell you that patients don't come in with their prescriptions at a steady pace. It tends to be either a feast or a famine. If I was a conspiracy theorist, I would suspect that patients waited outside my pharmacy until there was at least 6 of them, then they all come in together. Maybe I should check outside my door to see if someone has put up a sign saying "queue here until there is at least 6 of you." So in practice you dispense zero prescriptions for 10 minutes, then have to dispense 10 prescriptions in the next 10 minutes. No one likes to have to wait for their prescription, so this puts pressure on pharmacists to dispense faster.

Administration Comes Before Patient Care

In the four minutes (or less) that a pharmacist gets to dispense a medicine, they have to check the prescription is valid according to all the Ministry of Health criteria. They have to determine if the medicine is appropriate for the patient for whom it has been ordered, and they have to take care of any administrative tasks. In my pharmacy, I train new pharmacists who have just finished their pharmacy degree at University. As part of their training, they are required to produce a dispensing checklist. This is supposed to be a practical checklist of things they need to do before the patient leaves the pharmacy with their medicine. This checklist often runs to several pages long. This includes checking things like whether the patient details are correct, is the medicine suitable for this patient, is the form of medicine suitable for this patient, are there any interactions with other medicines the patient may be taking, etc. It is a complex set of tasks that requires a thorough process to ensure it is right.

Conveyor Belt Medicine

So in practice we end up with what I call "conveyor belt medicine." In other words, in the pursuit of efficiency we dumb down all the intellectual tasks so that we can just get the prescription out the door as quickly as possible. I have often thought of running a survey of my pharmacy patients asking if they would rather:
   a. get their prescription off the "conveyor belt" in 10 minutes, or
   b. wait for 15 minutes, but be assured that the pharmacist has time to discuss with you the consequence of this medicine and what you need to do to ensure best health.
I know which one I would prefer.

Warning! You Must Read This Entire Book Before Getting Your Next Prescription

I see patients at each end of the health spectrum. From patients with minor illness who come in to my pharmacy for some advice, right through to patients who are referred to my nutrition medicine clinic because they are so sick they have had to give up their work and their favourite activities.

While I love helping these very sick people and getting them back to a normal enjoyable life, I am often a little annoyed too. I'm annoyed because these people should never have been allowed to get this sick. I am also a little ashamed as I think of the number of patients that I have let leave my pharmacy without trying to educate them about how they can ensure optimal health. But not anymore, not on my watch!

Let me tell you about one of my current patients with irritable bowel syndrome. She is so sick that she reacts to almost every food. She is "surviving" on lamb and pears and nothing much else. This patient has a history of being treated for minor gastrointestinal upsets throughout her life. She was never told about how taking medicines to treat the symptoms of her condition could damage her gastrointestinal system more.

Now we have a long battle to reverse the changes because she has become very reactive to many of the treatments that we would normally use. For her it will also be a long and expensive battle, as we have had to get special formulations made just for her. This particular patient travels about 100km to see me, so she was not one of my local pharmacy clients. This is why I have written this book.

Another case involves a family that come to my pharmacy for their prescriptions. The mother of the family died last year in her late 60s. Far too young for anyone to die I might add. Anyway, before she died she was taking 18 different prescription medicines. We used to put her medicines in a blister pack so that she could co-ordinate taking such a large number of medicines. You can imagine that all my pharmacists used to run for cover when it was time to make her blister packs up!

Now the two adult daughters also come into my pharmacy. One has fairly robust health and usually only comes to collect the prescriptions for other members of the family. The other daughter seems to be following in her mum's footsteps. She is only in her 30s, but she is already taking 13 medicines. It is frustrating to see this young lady heading down a path of worsening health and decreasing quality of life. I know that spending some extra time and money on testing and treatments, which might be "outside the square" of conventional medicine, could result in a much more favourable outcome for her.

So my plea to you is read this book before you get your next prescription. The information in it could make a dramatic difference to your health and vitality.

2

Health Models:
The Pharmaceutical Industry Versus
The Natural Health Industry

A Suggestion For The Impatient Patient

The next three chapters provide some useful information as to how the health system is set up to ensure a cycle of increasing ill health. I think it is important that you understand how this has happened.

However, if you like to stampede through to the nitty gritty of learning the practical things you can do to improve your health, then you may want to skip ahead to chapter 5. But if you do skip ahead, please come back and read these next few chapters so that you can understand my entire message.

The Unnecessary Battle: Conventional Medicine
Versus Nutritional Medicine

It makes me angry! It drives me mad when I hear health practitioners criticizing the recommendations of other types of health solutions when they really don't know much about them. The attitude of "my way is the only way" is very closed minded. This is especially frustrating since I don't know any health professional who can claim to have all the answers.

I am sure that all health practitioners have the goal of making their patients well. That is something that doctors, nurses, pharmacists, physiotherapists, naturopaths, chiropractors and all other health practitioners have in common. But different groups of health practitioners have different approaches to the way they go about treating patients. The main difference between the pharmaceutical and natural health industries lies in how they develop solutions to health problems.

The Precise Pharmaceutical Industry

The pharmaceutical industry tends to try and develop medicines that act on very specific parts of metabolic pathways. They generally purify and isolate the active substance right down to the most specific chemical substance that provides the desired effects. This facilitates the production of incredibly powerful substances that block or stimulate a single chemical reaction in the body. In other words, it is a "one substance has one effect" type of model. This is great for some diseases, but for a lot of health problems things just aren't that simple.

In fact, how the human body works is very complicated. If you intervene at one step in a metabolic pathway, you are likely to cause an effect in another part of this or a different metabolic pathway. Or you try to switch a chemical reaction off, but instead the body has a feedback loop that makes the reaction go even faster, so you end up with the opposite effect to the one you were trying to create! Have you ever given an antihistamine to a child and expected them to get sleepy, only for them to get hyperactive and start jumping off the walls? It is incredibly complex and sometimes seems a bit illogical.

As an example, think of a flowing river that runs through a farmer's paddock. If he wants to stop the river flowing through that paddock, he could stick a great big boulder in the river further upstream. This would then stop the water flowing through his paddock, so the problem is solved. However, if the water can't flow through the paddock, it must start to flow somewhere else. It is likely that it will start to spring forth in other paddocks, or perhaps the buildup of pressure will eventually wash the boulder away causing the paddock to be totally flooded. Not such a smart solution after all. What would have been a better solution would have been to turn off the flow of water at the source. In that way, the river would stop flowing through the paddock and there would be no side effects from the excess water spilling over.

Well this is what can sometimes happen when you use a prescription medicine to completely block a metabolic pathway. You often get unintended effects in other metabolic pathways, which may cause health problems.

Staying Closer To Nature

On the other hand, many natural health solutions are developed using the original substance found in nature. In this way, they often have some of the effects that the drug might have, but being closer to nature are less likely to have some of the adverse effects of the more powerful drugs. That is a big difference.

Take for example a commonly used group of medicines called the statins. These drugs are used to lower cholesterol and prevent cardiovascular disease by blocking an enzyme called HMGCoA Reductase (believe it or not, it's full name is even longer). This enzyme controls a key step in the process in your body that makes cholesterol. So if you block this enzyme, you block your production of cholesterol. Sounds good doesn't it?

However, this pathway also makes a number of other substances that are important to health including coenzyme Q10, which is a vital nutrient needed by your body to make energy. So by blocking cholesterol, you also block energy production.

These statin drugs were developed from a natural substance called red yeast rice. Studies on red yeast rice have shown that it has many of the benefits of the statin drugs in terms of lowering cholesterol, but is less likely to have many of the side effects of these medications.

An Adjustable Valve Compared With A Sledge Hammer

Staying with the cholesterol example, magnesium has been shown to moderate the activity of the HMGCoA Reductase enzyme. So unlike the statin drugs that totally block this enzyme, magnesium acts more like a valve to slow it down or speed it up depending on what the body needs. So if the body needs more cholesterol (for example if you need more hormones), it will speed up the enzyme, but if the body needs less cholesterol, it will slow this enzyme down. This is a great illustration of the difference between the very potent and absolute effects of a drug compared with the more gentle and balancing effects of a nutrient. By the way, my research indicates that many people are deficient in magnesium!

Small Changes Can Make Huge Differences

There are also many examples of changing a natural substance, even only slightly, and getting great differences in actions in the body. Our hormones are one good example of this. No pharmaceutical company can patent a natural substance like a hormone. To enable them to patent a substance and therefore make a financial return on their research and development costs, they will make slight changes to the chemical structures of the hormone to create a unique substance. They test lots of different versions until they come up with one that has similar effects in the body to the natural hormone. But while the main effects can be similar, the side effects can sometimes be vastly different.

The natural hormone progesterone is an example of this. The synthetic progestins are copy drugs of the natural hormone progesterone. They have similar therapeutic effects to natural progesterone in terms of reducing the growth of cells and increasing their differentiation or development. So for women they work well to calm down menstrual cycle problems. However, the side effect profiles are very different as shown in table I.

Table I. Comparison of the effects of natural progesterone and synthetic progestins (from Dr John Lee, *What Your Doctor May Not Tell You About Menopause*, 2004).

Condition	Natural Progesterone	Synthetic Progestins
Water, mineral and electrolyte imbalance		✓
Depression		✓
Birth defect risks		✓
More body hair, thinner scalp hair		✓
Embolism risk		✓
Decreased glucose tolerance		✓
Allergic reactions		✓
Cholestatic jaundice risk		✓
Acne, skin rashes		✓
Protection against endometrial cancer	✓	✓
Protection against breast cancer	✓	
Normalises libido	✓	
Improves cholesterol profile	✓	
Improves new bone formation	✓	modestly
Improves sleep patterns	✓	

Everyone Is Different

Another key difference between the pharmaceutical industry and the natural health industry is the way the respective practitioners work. In particular, they tend to differ when it comes to their views on a concept that I refer to as biochemical individuality. What this concept of biochemical individuality means is that everyone is different in the way that they react to the environment, food and medicines.

So conventional medical practitioners work under the guidelines of "evidence-based medicine." This evidence-based approach seems great, since before a medicine can be used, the evidence must be fully evaluated and the medicine must prove it has benefits over and above its risks or side effects. The downside of evidence-based medicine is that the evidence is based on what happens when you treat large groups of the population. This population-based strategy ensures that the majority of people will get the desired effects. This is great if you are average or normal.

The Problem With Evidence-Based Medicine

Biochemical individuality means that some people are just a bit different. They do not react like the normal range of people so they might get stronger effects or weaker effects, and even sometimes completely different effects, which can lead to side effects or toxicity.

It is hard for conventional medical practitioners to understand patients who are not "normal." After all, the evidence says that this drug will help them, but this person complains they feel worse. If not handled properly, the patient can begin to feel less confident in their medical practitioner. In fact, this can often lead to feelings of frustration on behalf of the practitioner and the patient. This is usually the stimulus for a patient to start searching for alternative solutions from complementary health practitioners, or from the Internet. I have found that in general, natural health practitioners are taught to treat each person as an individual and tailor their treatment based on what they see for that individual.

Plus there are the time constraints that conventional medical practitioners work under. It is very hard to treat each patient as an individual and develop a treatment plan inside 10 minutes! By necessity, they must rely on pre-prepared treatment guidelines.

So who has the right answer? Are doctors, pharmacists and the pharmaceutical industry correct, or do complementary health practitioners have the answer?

I don't think there is a right or wrong answer. A lot of the things that conventional doctors and pharmacists do with support from the pharmaceutical industry are really great, particularly for acute illnesses. Conventional medical practice provides many patients with relief from suffering, or sometimes they simply provide reassurance that there is nothing seriously wrong with the patient. This can provide the patient with confidence that they can work on their diet or exercise to enable them to start to feel truly well.

There Is No "I" In Team

Similarly, many patients have received relief from the suffering of a long lasting medical condition with the help of complementary health practitioners. My view is that for the best results, conventional and complementary health practitioners should work together as a team. Unfortunately, examples of this form of team work in the health industry are not common. In fact, most health practitioners who do work in teams tend to work with practitioners with a similar skill base. For example doctors clump together in a medical practice or Naturopaths work together in a natural health clinic. Despite the fact that these health practitioners have the best of intentions, sometimes I feel they miss the point. They often will be treating the end signs or symptoms of a disease rather than treating the initial underlying metabolic dysfunction.

The Dodgy Mechanic

To illustrate this point in an extreme way, think about what you would do if an engine warning light came on in your car. You would likely take it to a mechanic and ask them to fix it.

What if when you got the car back you discovered that they fixed it by cutting the wire to the warning light. The immediate symptom has been relieved in that you can't see the warning light anymore. But the engine problem will only be getting worse. Depending on what that engine problem is, you might be able to continue to drive the car for another few months without any problems. But sooner or later, the problem will surface. Hopefully, not when you are half way across the Harbour Bridge in rush hour traffic!

So I guess it's not that anyone is wrong or right, or that one group has evil intentions and one group has good intentions. The approaches are often different and it would be nice to have a combined approach to get the best results for each individual patient.

A Lesson From My Favourite Movie

If you let me digress a little bit, I'll tell you about one of my favourite movies, called Nacho Libre. One of the main characters, Esqueleto, played by Hector Jimenez, says "I don't believe in God, I believe in science." The relevance of this quote to this chapter is amusing. It is not a case of whether or not we should believe in conventional or complementary medicine. We all know it's not either God or science. There is a place for both. Science is good and so is God or the universe or whatever force that is important to you. It is the same with natural health and conventional medicine. For the good of the patients there should be a mixture of both and they can work together in a complementary fashion to get the best health outcomes for individual patients.

Too Efficient For The Patient's Good

Another hurdle to good conventional medical practice is the time constraints doctors have to work within. When you go to see a doctor, they have to take a good history of what the problem is and what other problems from the patient's past may have lead to the problem, perform a physical examination if appropriate, prescribe laboratory tests if appropriate and decide on the most appropriate form of treatment, including prescriptions. All this is normally done in six to ten minutes. This model requires the doctor to use pre-prepared guidelines, or what we have previously mentioned as population-level, evidence-based medicine.

The Crime Scene: Gathering Evidence

However, unless the health condition is very simple, a lot more time is required to perform a proper analysis of the patient and really get to the cause of their health problems. In my clinical practice, I think of a patient's health and the problems that they are experiencing as a crime scene. You have got to be very meticulous and careful about gathering all the clues and putting them all together to find out what metabolic pathways might not be working properly. In other words, it takes time pouring over the crime scene to discover "who done it."

Have you ever watched a crime movie where they solve it in 10 minutes? No. They will bring in their forensic experts, examine the area for fingerprints or DNA, interview witnesses for more information, and interrogate the suspects. They will sweep through the crime scene in little tiny areas at a time until they can build up all those clues. So having the luxury of being able to take the time is another big part of good health care.

But There Are Bad Drugs, Right?

A lot of people are becoming nervous of taking drugs because of high profile mishaps like the pain killer Vioxx and the weight-loss drug Reductil which have been found to increase the risk of heart disease and stroke. People are a lot more questioning now about starting a new medicine.

I believe that there is no-one more motivated to see you achieve the best of health than you. For this reason, you should be cautious about any course of treatment that you intend to undertake. You need to talk to a range of trusted health professionals and seek out as much information as possible about the effectiveness and safety of any treatment before you start taking it. Having said that, the information on the safety of Vioxx and Reductil were not readily available when they first became available. In fact, the serious side effects only became known after statistical analysis of large quantities of data that was gathered after people started taking it. So it would be very difficult for you to have predicted the problems that these medicines would cause.

We have noticed in our pharmacy an increasing number of people that are getting nervous about taking medications. Often these patients ask me about the safety of a medicine, and I can usually reassure them that they are pretty safe, and that most of them work well when used as directed. But the human body is a very complex "machine" and we can never predict all the potential side effects. In other words, we cannot give a 100% guarantee that the medicine will be safe and effective.

Sometimes people have unique allergies to medications or the inactive additives in medicines. These allergies are unique to that particular patient and therefore will not have been seen in clinical trials. So there is no way of predicting such adverse effects for that person.

Less Is More Sometimes

So a sensible approach is to only use medications when absolutely necessary. We should only use medicines after we have spent time investigating what is happening in a patient's body. Because like the warning light on your car's dashboard, we do not want to mask minor symptoms of a serious disease.

However, in urgent situations there is often no time to ponder. For example, if you have had, or know of anyone who has had gallstones, you will know that they sometimes need injections of very strong pain killers as soon as possible to relieve the intense pain. It would be bad patient care to say to such a patient: "lets sit down for an hour and try and figure out why you are getting gallstones."

However, after the pain has gone, there is time then to consider why gallstones are forming in the first place, so that we can prevent further episodes.

Getting Careless With Common Medicines

From my experience as a pharmacist, I believe that we do overuse medicines. We tend to let down our guard and get a bit careless with medicines that we are very familiar with. A good example of this is our use of the pain relief medicines.

Paracetamol is a very commonly used painkiller and it is generally considered to be pretty safe as long as it's used in the right dosages. Certainly in the case of overdose and overuse, it can cause serious health issues such as liver problems. But even at lower doses we know that paracetamol can interfere with the production of an important enzyme in the body called glutathione peroxidase. This enzyme is important to clean up all the oxidative damage inside your cells in your body. So by taking paracetamol regularly, you can get a reduction in that important enzyme, which can lead to problems in the body.

There are also problems with the anti-inflammatory painkillers. They can have very strong effects on your digestive function. The flow on effects from an injured digestive system can affect all your body processes (but more on that in chapter 5). These medicines can also very quickly damage the kidneys, especially in older people.

Most older people that I try and talk out of taking these ant-inflammatory pain killers are surprised to hear that their

19

kidneys can be significantly damaged within weeks of taking these medicines.

Balancing Risks And Benefits

As a registered pharmacist I've got a good understanding of the way drugs work, both the good and the bad. I also have a healthy skepticism about the benefits as well as the risks. Generally on balance, the benefits do outweigh the risks. And if you understand the risks of your medicines there are often things you can do to reduce those risks and increase the chances of the best possible health outcome.

Speaking of reducing the risks, when I was a teenager I wanted to get a motorbike. My parents tried to educate me about the increased risks of a motorbike compared to a car. In fact, they made me go to a defensive driving course before they would let me buy a motorbike. At the course we talked about how the risks of dying from a motorbike accident were about the same as the risks of dying if you were a soldier in the infantry during World War I. That was certainly a sobering statistic. But they went on to educate me about how to reduce those risks by wearing visible clothing, protective helmet, gloves and boots, and by riding carefully. I made it through my teenage years with all my teeth, fingers and toes intact. And I guess that is a key message of this book: ask your trusted health professional how you can reduce your risks of medication-related adverse effects.

Natural Does NOT Mean Safe

Many patients self-medicate with drugs or herbal and nutritional supplements that they get from neighbours or family members. The assumption is that it is okay if they are natural.

It is a common misconception that if it's natural, it's good for you. A lot of the herbs are as potent as drugs. They're just the natural form of a drug in many cases. Some of the most toxic chemicals known are natural. Consider the organo-phosphate insect killers. They are natural but pretty deadly, especially if you're a fly. So as mentioned in the previous section which considered getting careless about the power of prescription medicines, you need to be very, very careful with natural substances too. It doesn't matter if it is a prescription medicine, a herb, a vitamin or a mineral supplement. Even energy-based treatments like homeopathic remedies, which are very safe, can cause problems if you take them without some expert guidance.

It's a bit like crossing a motorway blind. You might get across all right, but chances are you are going to get hit by a bus or a car. So it's always worthwhile getting some expert help and advice just to make sure you are going on the right track and not doing any harm.

Is A Combination Of Drugs And Nutrients Best?

Having studied pharmacy and nutrition medicine gives me a unique appreciation of the role of drugs and nutrients in health. While there are other dimensions to health, combining medica-tions and good nutrition has produced fantastic improvements in the health of most of the patients that I see in my Nutrition Medicine Clinic.

A good diet is core to getting good nutrients to start with. Most people I talk to claim they eat a healthy diet. Only occasionally do people say they eat a bad diet, and usually these people have a shockingly bad diet! You would not believe some of the stories I have heard. When I actually question people about their "good diet" they commonly eat a high calorie, low nutrient diet. It may not include takeaway food every day, but it is certainly not healthy. So good diet advice and education is well needed. Sometimes people need extra nutrient supplemen-tation with vitamins and minerals.

When A Good Diet Is Not Enough

While a good diet is the most important aspect of ensuring good health, sometimes people need a little bit extra. I personally try and eat a good diet, and strive to ensure that my meals and snacks are balanced and full of nutrients. Yet despite knowing what I should do, there are occasions when I slip up and eat something not so great for me. Like when my wife has just taken a batch of cheese scones out of the oven (I'm supposed to be dairy-free). A man can only resist so much temptation!

Anyway, even if we assume that we all eat a great diet 100% of the time, there are a number of other reasons why you might need to also take supplements. I've included these in an appendix at the back rather than take up all the space in this chapter.

Beyond Nutrition

There is a lot of research in other important health-related fields such as in mind medicine, energy medicine and structural alignment. While these modalities are really important, they are beyond the scope of this book. In this book we are focusing mainly on the prescription medicines and how they interact with nutrients, and how to use this knowledge to improve your health. So there is a lot of information that we don't know at the moment. However, if you are going to take a prescription medicine, understand how it affects your nutrient status so that you can ensure your best health in the future.

3

The Importance Of Nutrition

Do You Want Fries With That?

As part of educating people about how to achieve the best health from their prescriptions, the pharmacists in my pharmacy will sometimes recommend supplements that can enhance the effectiveness or reduce the side effects of a prescription medicine.

If your pharmacist recommends you take a supplement alongside your prescription without educating you about why that is important, then I guess you would naturally think they are just trying to sell you "fries with your burger."

It's A Matter Of Trust

The pharmacists in my pharmacy are carefully selected, not only on their clinical skills, but because they are caring and compassionate people. They genuinely care about the health of our clients, many of whom become friends and not just customers.

People choose to put their trust in our pharmacy because they know we care about them and respect them. They also know that we are continuously learning so we know all we possibly can about our health products and services. We consider it our professional responsibility to make sure our customers get the best health outcomes from their prescriptions.

Our pharmacists and support staff are not just pill counters.

Their role is to make sure you understand what is important to your health, and then it's up to you to decide what you do with the information you've been given. That comes down to the level of trust you have in your pharmacist, which is vital. At the end of the day, if you don't trust your pharmacist and are suspicious about their motives, then it is probably time to get another one. How well does your pharmacist stack up?

The Health Professional You See Most Often

Remember the old television commercials about your pharmacist being the "health professional you see most often." It is important then to make sure your pharmacist knows about the interactions of medicines and nutrients and is easy to communicate with.

So if your pharmacist does not provide you with information about what you need to do to ensure best health, then I would suggest they either don't care about your health, or they haven't kept up with the latest research about your medicines and your health.

Russian Roulette

So if you are not getting the extra special care that my pharmacists provide you may as well be playing Russian roulette. It is like you have a gun to your head and only one of the six chambers contains a bullet. In this game you have a one in six chance of the gun going off when you pull the trigger. In other words, you may take your prescription and get away without any side effects or disruption to core body processes. But maybe there is a major side effect that is going to cause you a lot of problems.

Our view is that it is better to prevent these problems in the first instance than to try and treat them once they have developed. Why take the gamble?

If Supplements Were Important, Wouldn't My Doctor Have Recommended Them On My Prescription?

Some doctors always prescribe appropriate supplements along-side the patients' prescription medicines. Other doctors don't necessarily prescribe these supplements as they have confidence that the pharmacist is best trained to help the patient get the best health outcomes from their prescription. There are some other doctors that haven't kept up with the research in the field of nutrition medicine, and these doctors might be defensive about their lack of knowledge and state that there is no evidence that the supplements are important. What they are really saying is that they are unaware of any evidence. To be honest, that is not really the fault of those doctors, since this information is not taught in a co-ordinated direct fashion at medical school.

To be familiar and comfortable with the effects of drugs on nutrients, doctors would have needed to undertake extra study in this ever developing field. Fortunately for the health of our patients, we are seeing more doctors in the former categories than in the latter.

Key Nutrients That Doctors Prescribe

In fact, most doctors will prescribe from a basic list of nutrients when needed. In the hospital setting, there is research being done on the use of a more comprehensive list of nutrients.

In our pharmacy, we are actively involved in training new pharmacists. It was interesting to learn from an intern pharma-cist who had been working in one of our major hospitals that they will now use probiotics in patients with diarrhoea as a safer alternative to common medicines. Generally what happens in hospital practice will gradually filter out into general practice. Sometimes it just takes a while for the information to become commonly used.

There are several nutrients that doctors currently working

in general practice will use regularly. One of the most common minerals and vitamins that they prescribe is iron. The understanding of the vital role of iron in maintaining health is well established in the medical profession. Most people understand the effects of iron deficiency on tiredness and the immune system. Folic acid is now prescribed regularly for women planning to become pregnant, as it is important for preventing neural tube defects in the new baby. Other commonly prescribed nutrients that we see in our pharmacy are the B-vitamins, multivitamins, and minerals such as magnesium and calcium.

Welcome Back Iodine

Recently we are seeing doctors prescribing iodine, which we haven't seen for a number of years. We know that iodine is deficient in the soils in New Zealand and the Government made the decision a long time ago to fortify salt with iodine. But of course many people now avoid salt, so we are seeing a lot of people coming through with iodine deficiencies, which is really fascinating.

Cost Is An Issue

But I guess apart from those main nutrients listed above, most are not funded. This means that a patient would have to pay the full cost for them. Doctors are sometimes reluctant to prescribe things that will put another cost on to the patient. However, if it is really important for your health, then at least you need to be aware of it and you can make that decision for yourself whether the benefits justify the costs.

What are the costs of not staying well? For example, if you were taking an antibiotic for a chest infection and then had to take a day off work because of diarrhoea, what would that cost you? Or if you were taking cholesterol medications and had reduced energy levels that meant you were too tired to go out with your friends and family, or didn't have the energy to tend to your vegetable garden. How would that make you feel? These are issues that you need to consider for yourself.

What Do Doctors Truly Think About Nutrition?

When I first started studying nutrition medicine one of my first assignments required us to interview a range of doctors about their view on the role of nutrition for health. All the responses I received were really positive about nutrition being vitally important for health. So doctors as a group tend to believe nutrition is very important for health.

However, in practice most doctors simply do not get enough time with patients to truly analyse and improve their diets. Plus it is quite specialist work. That's a bit like how dentistry has become a very separate part of medicine. Nutrition is not taught thoroughly at medical school or in pharmacy school. This is why I have undertaken years of extra training and education to acquire those skills so I can help patients better in this vital health area.

The Time-Poor Health System

We have mentioned how doctors don't have much time. Your doctor has approximately 10 minutes with you. It takes considerably more time than this to set a patient up with a proper diet that takes into account what metabolic pathways may not be working properly and what minerals and vitamins are essential to make that pathway work again.

Since this knowledge is not part of the core training at medical school, to help patients with nutrition would require that a doctor do a lot of research. That is why having a nutrition medicine expert helping you to sort those issues out can really be helpful.

Expensive Urine

Ever heard someone say that vitamins are just expensive urine? If that were the case then doctors would not prescribe iron, folic acid, magnesium and calcium. Ask anyone who is deficient in vitamin B12 how they feel after their injection and they will tell you it's like a turbo boost!

Some vitamins will colour the urine. Vitamin B2, for example, is a very bright yellow substance and so are the compounds that it is metabolized to before it is excreted in the urine. This is why when you take a supplement of B vitamins your urine turns yellow.

Even some drugs will colour the urine. For example, the drug rifampicin, which has been used in the past for tuberculosis, colours urine red. It's just a fact that it's metabolites are red. So that doesn't mean to say you're urinating out the rifampicin without any benefits. It just means that the metabolites that are excreted in the urine are coloured red.

Serious Medical Conditions Need Serious Drugs

Some people will think that nutrients are not as strong as drugs. Generally, nutrients are not as specific as drugs and their effects on particular metabolic pathways in the body are not as dramatic. But did you know that 70% of the causes of death are related to poor nutrition?

Which means that if you improved what you ate, you would have less risk of death from heart attacks, less stroke, less diabetes and less cancer. You would also be less likely to get one of the diseases that decrease your quality of life, such as arthritis, eczema, asthma, gout and many others.

In other words, if you could achieve ideal nutrient status, you would live a longer, disease-free life. Now even as a pharmacist, I don't know of any drug that can achieve that result. So perhaps that means that good nutrition is more powerful than good medicines!

Diet Is Most Important

Good nutrition starts with diet. It is not only what we decide to eat, but it also depends on what is in the foods we eat. Poor food choices and poor food quality (i.e. grown in mineral deficient soils) will increase our need for nutrient supplementation. Also, if we have any extra special nutrient requirements then we may also need extra nutrient supplementation.

Our nutrient requirements go up for many reasons including if we start doing exercise, if we are under stress, or during pregnancy. Some medications have side effects that cause nutrient depletions, so supplementation is required when taking these medications. So there is a whole number of factors that can affect nutrient status and therefore, our health.

There have been studies that show in people with type 2 diabetes, diet changes can improve their condition so much that they can actually stop all their diabetes medications. It reverses the disease process.

Need more convincing? Well, fish oils reduce the risk of death following a heart attack by 50%. These sorts of benefits are a lot more powerful than what is normally achievable with drugs. So nutritional interventions can provide incredibly powerful effects and help you achieve great health.

The Veterinarians Know About Nutrition

Interestingly, a lot of what we know about nutrition and health comes from the veterinary industry. It makes sense that if you have a prize bull, or a champion horse, you are going to make sure that they get the best nutrition. Even the productivity of a plain old dairy cow depends on the mineral content of the soil. And farmers go to great trouble and expense to make sure they analyse their soil so they can get the best yields from their cows or crops.

This doesn't mean there is no place for drugs. They are both important. The point I am keen to convey is that it's about

29

truly understanding what is happening in your body and choosing whatever intervention is best for you at that time. I don't think one is particularly stronger than the other, they all have their place.

How Come I Eat A Great Diet And I'm Still Sick?

I get a lot of my patients who tell me in their first interview "Oh, I eat a good diet." But is it really good? A lot of people consider a good diet is the fact that they don't eat takeaways very often. In other words, they say "Well, I don't eat fish and chips every night, so therefore I've got a healthy diet." When I actually analyze diets, which takes a lot of time and effort, we often see several imbalances in the intake of their macronutrients. And by that, I mean the balance of their proteins and their fats and their carbohydrates is wrong. As previously mentioned, this can have dramatic effects on health.

Jamie Oliver Gets The Publicity

Celebrity chef Jamie Oliver has examined what children are eating, including all the pre-prepared foods that are available in the supermarket. It is quite scary when the content of prepackaged foods is revealed; what they are supposed to have in them and what they do have in them are often surprisingly different. There can be a downside to the busy modern lifestyle which encourages the use of convenience foods to enable the preparation of meals very quickly for their family.

Are Your Veges All They Are Supposed To Be?

But even if you do manage to use wholesome fresh vegetables in your meals, how sure are you that it was grown in a soil that contains a full set of the nutrients that you need. I have already mentioned in a previous chapter about the iodine deficiencies in New Zealand soils. Our soils are also deficient in selenium, and through over-farming there can be magnesium deficiencies. There are a lot of reasons why the level of nutrients inside your food might not be as good as what they should be.

There are also particular conditions or diseases that may increase your requirements for vitamins, minerals and other nutrients. For example, in pregnancy, the need for protein and omega-3 fatty acids goes up dramatically. This is a problem for many women because they often feel nauseous and eat less than normal rather than more.

Genetic Polymorphism – Why I Am Unique

Some people have changes in their genes that can affect how their body functions. These are not full-blown genetic defects like Down's Syndrome, but are only minor changes, which are termed genetic polymorphisms.

So how could this affect you? Well let's say, for example, you have a polymorphic change in an enzyme that needs zinc to make it work properly. A good example is the enzyme that metabolises fats from your diet (delta-6-desaturase, or d6d for short). This means that for this enzyme to work properly, you need to have a lot more zinc than a "normal" person. So what this means for you is that if you have a good diet containing a normal level of zinc in it you won't break down your fats. This could result in an inflammatory condition, such as arthritis, or brain problems or even heart problems, as the joints, brain and heart all require the good fats to work properly.

But by taking extra doses of zinc, the enzyme begins to function and your health problems will improve. This is an example whereby taking the recommended daily allowance of zinc is not enough. In other words, it supports the concept we discussed earlier called biochemical individuality, which means that everyone is different. Some people need more nutrients and so a "one-size fits all" model doesn't work.

Good Health Versus The Absence Of Disease

I see a lot of people in my pharmacy and in my clinic. My clinic patients are often very sick patients that get referred to me for intensive evaluation and treatment. In contrast, most of my pharmacy clients often consider themselves as "well." I often enquire about how they're feeling, and once you get past the "good thanks" polite answer and they realize that you are genuinely interested in their health they often mention tiredness or aches and pains that they shrug off as just being due to getting older, or being under a lot of stress at work.

A Common Story

A common story goes something like this: "I do like to have a nap on the couch during the day to recharge my batteries. And its not unusual for me to fall asleep at 7 o'clock while I'm watching tele in the evening. But I am getting older and I do work really hard, so that is to be expected." While tiredness and aches and pains may be quite common, it's not healthy and it's not to be expected. We should be able to cope with a full day's work and still be able to interact with our family in the evening. We should be able to do a reasonable day's work even as we get older.

Losing the ability of our muscles to work properly and effectively is not a consequence of healthy ageing. It is a consequence of poor nutrition. It just happens that the effects of poor nutrition add up over time. So it appears as though these problems are associated with normal age-related changes. But, if we can keep the right nutrients going into bodies we can stay mentally alert and we can stay physically active.

For a lot of people the deterioration in their wellness and

vitality is a gradual process so they don't really notice it. For some nutrients you can reverse the deficiency very quickly which gives people a "wow" reaction. For other nutrients, it takes time for them to be incorporated into the various body systems, so the improvement in health and vitality is more gradual.

A common cause of unhealthy ageing is poor diet, which can lead to inflammation in the gut, which in turn reduces the absorption of nutrients from food. The nutrient deficiency can interfere with hormone production, and hormones have a strong impact on how you feel. Most changes in hormone balance result in lower muscle bulk.

We all know the examples of some of the cheats in the body-building world that use steroids to increase their muscle bulk. The steroids are like hormones, so low levels of hormones will certainly make you the opposite of a bodybuilder.

The production of energy in the body is well researched. It involves many different nutrients and vitamins. It is not surprising then that tiredness or reductions of energy levels are a key sign of nutrient depletion. A lot of people think that they don't have a disease, but they certainly are not functioning at an effective and well level. That is the difference between an absence of disease and true wellness. If you are well, you will have an abundance of energy.

> I have put an "Optimal Wellness Diet" on
> the resources pages of my website.
> I encourage you to visit the resources pages at
> www.OptimalPrescriptionHealth.co.nz/resources
> and download a copy for yourself.

4

Martin's Story

What Made A Pharmacist Start Looking Outside Conventional Medicine And Become A Nutrition Medicine Expert?

I am not really sure why I was drawn to the pharmacy profession. When I was growing up, my local pharmacy seemed like a nice place to be. It was filled with friendly staff and pleasant smells. The pharmacist was approachable and helpful. I always had an interest in health and I guess I had a yearning to understand how the body works and how drugs affect the body. I was also brought up to strive to make a positive contribution to society. So what better way than to become a pharmacist.

Then after many years of pharmacy practice it started to concern me that there was actually a lot of people who just didn't feel well, despite using the best conventional medicine had to offer. I also started to question why certain illnesses were so common.

In particular, I saw a lot of patients coming in to get antidepressants and particularly women in their 30s and 40s. That got me thinking, is there a hormonal cause of depression? Are there really that many women who are depressed or is some sort of hormone imbalance causing these issues for these women?

So I started doing some research into how hormones can affect the brain. A common thread that ran through a lot of this research was the importance of nutrition.

The Importance Of Nutrition Becomes Apparent

As I started to learn more about nutrition and the role of nutrients in the normal functioning of the human body, I started to think more and more about all the vitamins and supplements that we had in the pharmacy. I realized that we were not taught much about these vitamins and supplements at pharmacy school, and most of my knowledge had been picked up from reading educational materials from the vitamin companies.

That's when I came to the realization that I really needed to obtain some unbiased training in this field. After completing several courses in nutrition medicine, I attended a lecture by one of the leading nutrition medicine doctors from Australia. He happened to be a professor at a university that offered a nutrition medicine degree. He inspired me so much that day, that I enrolled in the degree and started my formal nutrition medicine education.

Now I get great reactions from my customers who come in to my pharmacy when we start talking about their health. I often get comments like "wow, you know so much about this stuff, you're not JUST a pharmacist are you?" That really makes my day, knowing that you have been able to truly help someone, rather than just relieve their symptoms.

The Blind Man And The Elephant

But the more I learn, the more I get an appreciation of how much more there is still to learn. It's a bit like the story of a blind man and the elephant. If the blind man grabs the elephant's tail, he will think that it is a small, thin, snake-like object.

It is not until he starts to move along the tail that he comes to the back legs of the elephant and starts to realize that there is a lot more to an elephant than a tail. It is actually one of the biggest animals on the planet.

As I started to learn more about the importance of nutrition in health, I realized I was only grasping the tail of the elephant. There was so much more to this science.

Have You Had Any Health Problems Yourself?

Like a lot of people, I do have my own tragic family health story. When my father was in his 20s he developed a very debilitating form of arthritis that has steadily progressed to steal much of his quality of life. Unfortunately, because there is a hereditary link, it can affect future generations. Indeed, my brothers and I have all been affected by this disease to some extent. So my dad and I share a common disease. It's called ankylosing spondylitis, which is a disease that affects the spine.

Ankylosing spondylitis is an arthritic disease, so all the vertebrae or the little joints in the spine will calcify and all the discs between the vertebrae will just collapse. So you end up with the person getting shorter and stooped and having no movement in their spine at all and that's certainly how my dad's disease has progressed.

He is now about 30 centimeters shorter than what he was as a young man. He has got absolutely no movement in the spine. He even has to twist on his seat to see what is beside him. It has really affected his quality of life in a big way, and to some extent, that disease is inheritable, which is why I've always tried to maintain a fairly active life in an attempt to prevent those disease changes happening to me.

The Wrong Thing To Do

When my dad was first diagnosed with ankylosing spondylitis he was told to rest and to use anti-inflammatory painkillers because the pain can be quite intense. Unfortunately, those two things can be quite detrimental to the long-term outcome for ankylosing spondylitis, which is why, I guess, my dad is now pretty much crippled and immobile. The risk is that by resting, the joints stop moving and seize up. Then the muscles get weaker and can't support the joints.

Furthermore, the anti-inflammatory medications that he took, which I will talk about in a later chapter, can disrupt gut function and cause more inflammation, which is one of the underlying factors that imbalance the immune system.

So How Has This Disease Affected Me

I have to admit that in my younger years, despite my training as a pharmacist, I didn't understand or know much about nutrition and supplementation, and so I was actually doing quite a lot of the wrong things and ended up with the same disease myself.

It is quite frightening that very little is taught about nutrition in medical school, despite the fact that the major diseases that can kill us are related to poor nutrition. So here I was, a fully qualified pharmacist with no idea that my diet was contributing to poor health.

Making Positive Choices

However, I was determined to take a different track from my dad. I saw the way he ended up physically and didn't want to get that way. My dad was a really good athlete in his younger years. Now, he cannot even kick a ball in the backyard with his grandkids and that's tragic.

I don't have any grandkids yet, but if I am blessed with grandchildren, I would love to be fit and healthy enough to teach them how to play a range of sports, whether I'm 50 or 80 years old!

I love playing with my kids, especially playing football with them. In fact, I'm playing football with my eldest son in a senior men's league this year, which has been real fun.

My Health Bombshell

When I was in my 30s I started getting intense back pain. This was diagnosed as ankylosing spondylitis by a rheumatologist. To avoid a tragic outcome for myself, I have changed my diet, treated my nutrient imbalances, and have stayed active physically. So far I have had greatly different health than my father had by my age. Now in my mid-40s, I have no back pain and no joint discomfort at all.

I hope my story can be inspiring to others. My dad and I are two men with a similar genetic makeup, with the same disease, but with completely different health outcomes. I attribute this difference to the different environment that we have been exposed to, mainly the different diet, activity levels and nutrient supplementation.

Has Ankylosing Spondylitis Impaired Your Quality Of Life Like It Did For Your Dad?

As I mentioned, I was first diagnosed with ankylosing spondylitis when I was in my 30s. I had a lot of sore backs, especially first thing in the morning. When I would get up in the morning I could hardly move, and I would look like a 90-year-old man shuffling down the hallway stooped over until I got warmed up. But there is an old saying: "what does not kill you makes you stronger." So in a way, I am grateful for having that disease because it's made me aware of my own health.

If I hadn't experienced the back pain, I would not have known that my diet was poor and therefore pushing me towards an early grave or significant illness. I would only have realized too late after years of damage had been done.

Now I consider my pain or inflammation as like a warning light on the car dashboard. When any sort of pain or inflammation comes up, I know that things are not well with my metabolism, and so I take heed of the warning and take action. I will then make improvements to my diet (because it's so easy to slip into bad habits), and may increase the dose of my nutrient supplements. I make sure I am getting enough exercise and my lifestyle is at an optimal level. And so I think now I'm actually much healthier because of my disease. I'm more aware of my health than I would have been if I had not developed this disease.

In other words, in turning my disease off, I have turned great health on.

What Have You Done That's Helped You?

In previous sections of the book I mentioned some of the health changes I have personally made. These include changes to my diet, essential nutrient supplementation, and changing the type of exercise that I do.

My Diet

The most dramatic changes have probably been my diet. As a pharmacist, we didn't really get any proper nutrition training. However, there is a lot of information encouraging us to cut the fat out of our diets. So in my quest to be healthy, I had a really low-fat diet, and thought I was going to live a long and healthy life.

But when you focus on cutting fat out of your diet, you have to replace it with something else. Like most people who listen to the "cut the fat" message, I ended up with a diet that was really high in inflammatory carbohydrates, especially those with a high glycemic index. As well as being high in inflammatory carbohydrates, my diet was very low in quality nutrients. So in my well-meaning but ignorant quest to be healthy, I was actually poisoning myself.

My diet is now pretty well balanced for macronutrients, including fats, protein, fibre and carbohydrates. Fat is not a dirty word for me anymore, in fact fats are essential for health.

I even take extra fat as a supplement! But you have to have the right balance of good fats in your diet, namely the trans versus cis unsaturated fats, the saturated versus unsaturated fats, and the omega-3 versus omega-6 unsaturated fatty acids.

Understanding all the different types of fat and the health benefits they provide is actually very complex. Some fats even interfere with the metabolism of others. So it would pay to talk to a suitably qualified health practitioner about how to optimize your fat intake.

Protein Is Good

The amount and the quality of the protein you eat is also important. My new diet includes a lot more high-quality protein. This is really important for muscle growth, the production of enzymes (which make everything in your body work), brain health and a number of other functions.

Balance Is Important

I have also changed the type of carbohydrates that I eat. Instead of highly refined grains, I now eat more vegetables. This means that I also get a great deal more vitamins and minerals from my food. There are also some specific anti-inflammatory foods, such as berries and fish, which I have incorporated into my diet.

Identifying My Poisons

One very important change I have made was to test for food allergies and sensitivities and to remove those foods from my diet. For me, those foods are gluten, dairy and cashews. I should issue a word of caution, that while the general principles of this diet are healthy, everyone is different. Therefore, this may not be the optimal diet for you.

Born To Run

From a lifestyle point of view, I don't do as much running as I used to, since this is a catabolic form of exercise. Catabolic means it breaks down body tissues more than it builds them up. I used to run marathons and at that time I had very low levels of body fat as you would expect. I still run regularly since this helps me play football better, but just nowhere near as far as I used to. Many of my runs are with Charlie my Labrador, who is not an endurance athlete (she's quite a chunky girl!) and just loves the shorter distance runs along the beach. So that suits us both just fine.

Preventing Frailty Starts In Your 40s

Instead of the two hour long runs I used to do as part of marathon training, I started doing a number of other forms of exercise that would help to build muscle mass. In other words, I started some weight training. Once you get over 40 the natural reduction or decline in hormone levels starts to take effect, which makes it harder to maintain your muscle mass. I figured that to maintain my vitality into old age, I needed to maintain my muscle mass now. That way, I am starting my journey into the later half of my life with a good baseline level of muscle.

I'm A Yoga Convert

I also took up yoga, which is great for stretching and staying supple. As I mentioned, my Dad has zero movement in many of his joints, so I have seen how debilitating that can be. I started practicing yoga so I could avoid losing my joint range of motion. What I did not know when I started practicing yoga was the effect that it can have on your mind. A good yoga teacher will guide you to free your mind and balance your whole perspective on life. I am very grateful for Denise at the Yoga Sanctuary for her wisdom and guidance in my yoga practice.

Avoiding Further Damage

I have avoided the pain-killing non-steroidal anti-inflammatory drugs (NSAIDs) that my Dad took because I know that they disrupt the gastrointestinal system. In the early days when my pain was really bad, I would occasionally take one just when needed. I don't believe you should suffer unnecessarily. Nowadays, I don't have any pain or inflammation so I haven't needed to take an anti-inflammatory pain killer for years. That is really helpful to avoid any gut dysfunction and therefore increased inflammation.

My Supplements

There are many nutrients that I have used over the years to reduce my inflammation and repair my metabolic pathways. Probably the most important area that I needed supplements for was my digestion, which was pretty poor. I explain in a later chapter how important digestion is to good health.

I have also used nutrients to balance my immune system. I remember back when my kids were young, I used to get every bug that they brought home. Now I consider that my immune system is like a shield of steel and I have not had a sick day off work in years.

Well that is my story. Through a combination of those five factors; diet, exercise, nutrient supplementation, avoiding disruptive medicines and improving digestion, I have turned off my ankylosing spondylitis. Plus I feel much better and think much clearer. To quote Jack Black from the movie Nacho Libre (please read with a Mexican accent): *"My life is good."*

5

Digestion:
The Core Of Your Health

Why Is Digestion So Important?

This comes to a phase of the book where I'm looking at individual body systems, medications and nutrients and what we can use specifically to improve our health. It is not by chance that digestion is the number one first body system that I review. Two thirds of adults have some form of irritable bowel symptoms.

A lot of people have digestive problems, and since digestion is the core of your health system this means that the majority of people are currently unwell or are on the way to becoming unwell. When I refer to digestive problems I'm talking about things like bowel upsets such as diarrhoea and constipation, as well as bloating, flatulence, heart burn, indigestion or even nausea and vomiting.

Gut Problems Affect Much More Than Just The Gut

While these symptoms are uncomfortable, many people don't consider them serious and just live with them. But remember the story of the warning light on the dashboard of your car. There are very important flow on effects from poor digestion in many other areas of your body including your immune system. Over 70% of your immune system resides in your gut. This makes sense, since you stick all sorts of foreign objects (food and drink) into your gut. So there needs to be a good defense mechanism to keep out the bad guys and allow the absorption of nutrients.

Inflammation is a key tool of the immune system, in that it helps to mobilize your army against any invaders. So you can see how inflammation is linked to poor gut function via the immune system. This is such an important concept for health that I'll repeat it:

Poor Digestion ⇨ Unbalanced Immune System ⇨ Inflammation ⇨ Disease

Inflammation involves pain, swelling, redness and heat in a damaged area. So following an injury to some part of the body, a good inflammatory process is essential to repair the damaged part of the body.

Unfortunately, when the gut is damaged, the immune system becomes unbalanced and inflammation can set in for the long term. Our beneficial defensive response (inflammation) then becomes disruptive. Once that happens, many other areas of the body can be affected, including close by areas such as the bowel (constipation or diarrhoea) and far away places such as the brain, lungs, joints, in fact any tissue at all. So I hope you can see why the gut is the core of good health.

I have created the following flow chart to show how essential the gut is in the causes of disease.

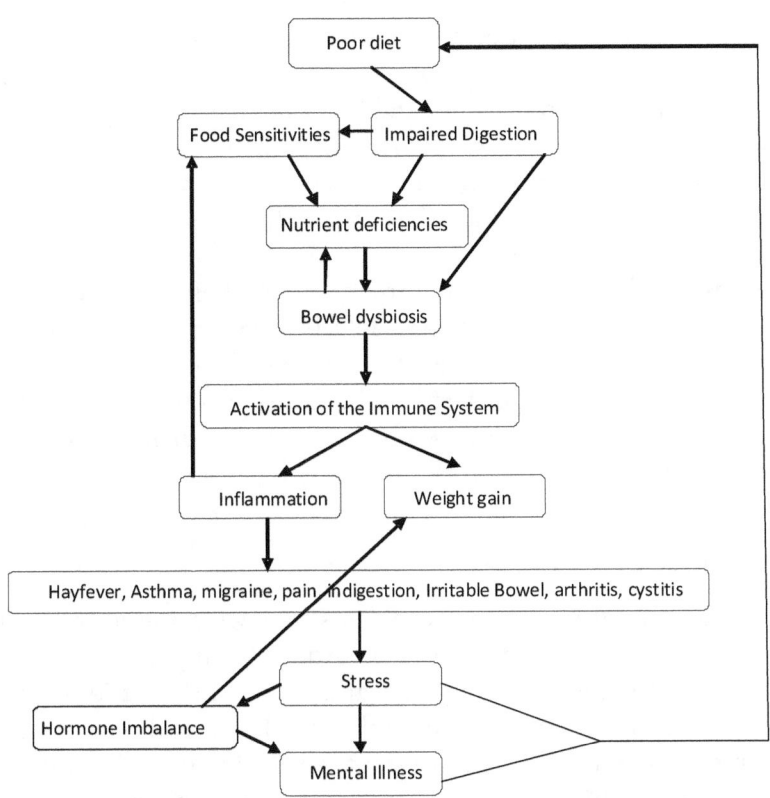

Digestion And Your Brain

We've mentioned that there are a number of ways that poor digestion can interfere with normal processes in the body. First, if your digestion is not working properly, you won't absorb the nutrients in your food properly. This includes protein, which contains amino acids. I think of proteins as a sentence, peptides are the words and the amino acids are the letters that make up the words that make up the sentences. So if you're not getting enough protein digested, you're not getting enough amino acids into your body.

The amino acids are important to make all the neurotransmitters in your brain. Neurotransmitters are the chemicals that run throughout your brain and elsewhere in the body. Their main role is in the brain where they help all your thought processes work, help your mood and assist with concentration. Similarly, the B vitamins are vitally important for brain function. There are studies that show anything from apathy, confusion, depression, right through to Alzheimer's disease are more likely if you are deficient in the B vitamins. So certainly not absorbing those nutrients can have an effect on depression.

There are also indirect effects of digestion on the brain. For example, if you have diarrhoea ten times a day, then the stress of that can affect your mood.

Digestion And Gout

So it is not surprising that problems in a wide variety of areas in the body are related to poor digestion. Gout is a disease that can affect the joints, mainly toes and ankles. In these joints you get a buildup of uric acid crystals, which are really sharp and therefore painful. The pain of gout is very intense. Contrary to conventional thinking, we find that the main problem in people who suffer from gout is not that they make more uric acid than anyone else. Instead, gout is a consequence of their metabolism being out of balance to start with.

Usually patients with gout have a diet that contains too much of the high glycemic index carbohydrates causing insulin resistance. That's like an early form of diabetes. This imbalance in metabolism causes the excretion of uric acid to be reduced. So if you are not getting rid of your uric acid, the levels build up, then they crystalise in joints and cause the pain of gout. However, this metabolic imbalance also causes extra weight gain around the belly region, which results in increased production of inflammatory chemicals in the body. This inflammation upsets digestion.

Therefore, gout is usually a warning sign that all those changes are taking place, which is why it's really important not just to take painkillers and treat the pain of gout, but to deal with all the causes.

If the cause is insulin resistance and you don't treat that, you're more likely to get diabetes. Once you get diabetes you're more likely then to get heart disease and eventually you become quite incapacitated. So again, it's a matter of treating the underlying condition rather than turning off the warning light.

What About Asthma, Can Poor Digestion Aggravate Asthma?

There are a number of studies that show that asthma is an inflammatory condition. We have talked before about the digestive core being responsible for moderating your production and release of inflammatory and anti-inflammatory chemicals. There are studies that show, for example, that the intake of key nutrients will dramatically change the risk of getting asthma. One of those key nutrients is fish oil. These studies have shown that if you have a diet that is deficient in fish oils, you have a 30% higher chance of getting asthma. So if you're not digesting your food properly, particularly your fats in this example, then you're at a much higher risk of asthma.

Also, if your whole gastrointestinal system is inflamed from eating the wrong foods, then that causes inflammatory chemicals to be released. More details on that are included in the chapter on asthma.

We have mentioned the importance to health of proteins being broken down to amino acids. Well if they don't get broken down by digestion, then the big undigested proteins can enter the bloodstream. Your blood does not ordinarily see these big proteins, so it doesn't recognize them as food. Instead, it thinks the proteins are a foreign object, which may be a dangerous threat. So it mobilizes its army to help kill off the "invaders." So the presence of whole proteins in the blood results in inflammatory cytokines running around in your body.

Now if your genetic makeup means you're predisposed to getting asthma, then these inflammatory cytokines will produce wheezing and respiratory hyper-responsiveness and all those things that cause asthma. So you can see how there is a direct effect on asthma from poor digestion.

What About The Immune System, Is That Affected By Poor Digestion?

Research shows that about 70% of the immune system resides in the gut. So you don't need to be a rocket scientist to see that anything that affects the gut will affect the immune system. If you've got poor gut function, you've got a poor immune system – simple as that.

A major part of the gut immune system is a protective lining called secretory immunoglobulin A. We mentioned previously the ability of proteins to cause immune system problems. To illustrate this point, think of your body as a house and your immune system as the security system. Now if you have lots of invaders (proteins) coming through the front door, your immune system is alerted and starts to protect the front door. It does this by locking the door, nailing up boards for extra strength, positioning additional security guards, fire-fighters and ambulance staff at the front door. In fact, the fire-fighters can spray water and foam around to reduce the risk of fire, which can create a big mess.

In the meantime, your back door is just wide open with no guard on it because all of your immune cells are at the front door. So in addition to being more susceptible to inflammatory disorders, you are also more likely to be susceptible to infection, for example from colds and flus. In other words, there is an imbalance of the immune system.

What medicines affect digestion?

Many medicines affect digestion. The most commonly pre-scribed medications in New Zealand are the proton pump inhibitors (known as PPIs), which are often prescribed for heart burn or reflux. Many people would know them by the names omeprazole (the most common one), but also pantoprazole and lansoprazole.

Mineral Deficiencies

The PPI medicines are very powerful at reducing stomach acid. So if you have heart burn or reflux, they can make the condition feel a lot better, since there is less acid in the stomach contents to burn, which sounds great. But they can actually be doing a lot of damage to your health in the meantime. Stomach acid is really important for digestion. It's important for acidifying all your minerals, so patients taking PPIs often get deficiencies of calcium and magnesium.

Stomach Sterilisation

Stomach acid is important to sterilize the stomach contents. This is quite a simple system whereby the high acid levels in the stomach kill any invading bugs or parasites that enter the stomach with your food.

Impaired Digestion

Stomach acid is also the trigger for the production of digestive enzymes in the pancreas which then flows into the small intestines. So if you don't have enough stomach acid, then you don't produce digestive enzymes. If you don't produce digestive enzymes, then you are not going to digest all your food and it will cause all those problems that we've listed above, such as nutrient deficiencies and immune system activation.

H2 Antagonists – The Little Brother Of PPIs

There are also drugs called the H2-antagonists, which have names like ranitidine and famotidine, that lower stomach acid. While they are not as strong as the proton pump inhibitors that we talked about, they certainly affect acid production in the stomach.

NSAIDs: Irritating Little Drugs

There are a number of drugs that just by their nature are quite irritating to the stomach lining. Medicines like the non-steroidal anti-inflammatory drugs (NSAIDs). You probably know them as anti-inflammatory painkillers such as ibuprofen and diclofenac, for example. They will physically irritate the gut lining, which interferes with the production of stomach acid. This will cause inflammation in the stomach. Inflammation of the gut lining is a common side effect of NSAIDs.

How Can I Test For Digestive Disruption?

There are a lot of quite complicated tests you can do, some of which are quite invasive, such as endoscopy, whereby they place a camera down into your stomach to observe any big changes in the appearance of the lining of your esophagus and stomach. Your doctor can talk to you about it if you have a lot of strong symptoms. These tests are not very pleasant.

If you have a lot of wind, burping or farting, if you get a lot of bloating after meals or tenderness, cramping in the stomach, diarrhoea or constipation, nausea or vomiting then it is likely that your digestion is impaired and you have some inflammation going on.

These symptoms are not present in normal healthy people. Sorry guys, but regular farting is not just stuff guys do, it is a sign that digestion is not healthy.

Treating Digestion Problems

Making the symptoms of indigestion go away is relatively easy. However, actually fixing the underlying problems in someone with poor digestion is a lot more complicated. In fact, just understanding the complex interaction of hormones and neuro-peptides that make the gut function is hard enough. So there is not a "one-size fits all" approach to treating digestive problems. Each patient is unique and in my clinic we tailor solutions especially for each patient.

Doing The Wrong Thing

Medications such as omeprazole, pantoprazole, lansoprazole and ranitidine are designed to reduce the amount of stomach acid that your body produces. However, most cases of heart burn are NOT caused by too much acid in the stomach.

Heart burn is caused by the valve at the top of the stomach not closing off properly, which means you are not able to keep your stomach acid in your stomach. There can be many causes of this, but the most common one is consumption of a diet that contains too many high glycemic index carbohydrates (i.e. too many sugary things). Often a change in diet will correct the underlying cause of the problem, and allow you to stop taking your medication. Sometimes you may also need some herbs to soothe the oesophagus to enable it to heal up while you are correcting the faulty valve at the top of the stomach.

"This All Sounds Too Hard, Why Don't I Just Take Omeprazole?"

Good question. If omeprazole had no side effects, and if a faulty valve at the top of the stomach caused no other health problems then I'd say continue to take omeprazole. But neither of these is true.

Think of the warning light on the car dashboard again. Well

if our diet is high in simple sugars, this increases your likelihood of a lot of other serious illnesses, especially diabetes and heart disease. So would you want to know if your diet is optimal or would you rather cover up the warning light?

Heart burn is also a sign of digestion not working properly, which can lead to nutrient deficiencies. If you have a lack of some nutrients many of your metabolic pathways won't work properly, leading to ill health in any number of areas. So heart burn is not just an inconvenient consequence of modern living, it is an early warning sign that should be thoroughly investigated.

Don't Ignore The Warning Signs:

Poor digestion can have an amazing impact on your long term health. If you don't feel 100% healthy in your gut, then you should take action. Poor digestion can lead to:

- Nutrient deficiencies, leading to:
  - Tiredness
  - Fatigue
  - Brain fog
  - Anxiety
  - Anemia
  - Allergies;
- Low immunity (more infections, colds and flus);
- Inflammatory conditions such as asthma, arthritis, eczema, heart disease;
- Irritable bowel syndrome (constipation and/or diarrhoea);
- Weight gain or weight loss;
- Many more health problems.

In fact, some health experts believe that poor digestion is one of the leading causes of disease.

Stomach Acid Is Not The Bad Guy!

The natural production of stomach acid declines as we get older. This is the first clue that stomach acid is actually one of the good guys. If it were bad, then many "acid-related diseases" would be more common in young people rather than in the elderly, which is obviously not the case. Stomach acid is essential for proper digestion of food into its key nutrients. Especially the breakdown of protein and minerals such as calcium and magnesium.

If you end up with a protein deficiency, then you really are going to suffer. Protein is important for producing:

- Muscle;
- Hormones;
- Neurotransmitters (brain chemicals); and
- Enzymes (which make all your metabolic pathways work efficiently).

Imagine having small weak muscles, hormone imbalances, a shortage of brain chemicals and sluggish metabolism. You obviously wouldn't be a highly performing person. At best you would be able to drag yourself through each day!

Stomach acid is an essential trigger that signals your body to produce digestive enzymes. So no acid, means no digestive enzymes. No digestive enzymes, means poor digestion of nutrients and all the problems described above.

Low Stomach Acid Can Cause Heartburn!

So if low stomach acid causes heartburn, why do medicines that lower stomach acid improve my heartburn? When you use PPIs to lower stomach acid, the reflux of stomach contents into the oesophagus still happens. But because it has no acid in it, it does not burn. However, the reflux still happens. The burning is relieved, but the underlying condition is not. In fact, as we have noted above, stomach acid performs a variety of vital functions in the body, so these medications often make your digestion worse. You feel better, but you are worse off!

When stomach acid is high, your body produces a number of hormones that actually signal the valve between the oesophagus and stomach to close off. So increasing stomach acid will encourage the faulty valve to work properly and actually stop heart burn.

So Just How Safe Is Omeprazole?

Like all medications, omeprazole has benefits and side effects. One of the side effects of omeprazole that has been proven include mineral deficiencies (especially calcium and magnesium). A lack of calcium and magnesium has been associated with:

- loss of bone,
- muscle cramping,
- high blood pressure,
- heart disease,
- cancer,
- anxiety,
- migraine,
- many other health problems.

Other common side effects of omeprazole include:
- headache,
- diarrhoea,
- constipation,
- nausea,
- abdominal pain and
- flatulence.

So if you need to take omeprazole, then you need to be vigilant for the side effects so you don't do yourself any long term harm.

If you are taking omeprazole for heart burn, then you owe it to yourself to identify the cause of the heart burn and put that right, and thereby be able to stop your omeprazole, ensuring the best health in the long term. But a note of caution, you should not stop taking any medication without talking to your doctor or pharmacist first. You may have a condition different to heart burn that does require you to stay on omeprazole. Plus, it is difficult to just stop taking omeprazole, since a flare-up of symptoms often happens. Sometimes you need to heal the lining of your gut, so that when you do stop taking omeprazole, you won't experience undue discomfort.

Lots Of People Take Omeprazole – It Must Be Safe

How many people do you know who take omeprazole and feel really well? I don't know many. My goal in providing this information for you is to educate you so that you can make informed choices about your health. What you do with this information is your own business.

There are a couple of tests that you can do yourself in the comfort of your own home to help determine whether or not you have enough stomach acid. Visit www.OptimalPrescriptionHealth.co.nz/resources to obtain your "Guidelines for the Self Testing of Stomach Acid."

6

Treating Heart Disease

My Friend Told Me That Cholesterol Drugs Were Bad For You. Should I Avoid Them?

One of the differences between conventional and complementary medicine that we discussed in the early chapters was the pressure for efficiency in the conventional medicine system. This pressure has resulted in the development of predetermined disease treatment guidelines. Your average doctor just doesn't have enough time to spend with each patient.

In contrast, complementary medicine views people as biochemically individual. That is, every person is different. So rather than asking if cholesterol medicines are bad, the more important question to ask is why is your cholesterol high? The answer will be different for different people.

Why Is My Cholesterol High?

There can be a number of reasons for raised cholesterol. What is going on in your body might be quite different to what is going on in your friend's body.

One reason for cholesterol levels to go up is as a protective mechanism. For example, if your body is under a lot of inflammatory stress, then cholesterol levels will rise. Another reason for cholesterol to go up relates to your hormone levels, since hormones are made from cholesterol. So if you have low levels of hormones, then your body will try and make more cholesterol. Your body will naturally put cholesterol levels up so you have more raw materials with which to make hormones from.

Middle Aged Men And Their Hormones

For example, a male in his 40s or 50s has probably got a decline in hormone function and that may be a reason why the body is putting up the cholesterol to try and boost his hormone levels back to healthy levels. So high cholesterol levels are definitely a marker for poor health. So it's important to treat it and especially its causes.

One important hormone for men is testosterone. A decline in testosterone is associated with lower muscle mass, grumpy mood, excessive sweating, low libido, and inability to think clearly. Sound like anyone you know?

Cholesterol-lowering medications have been shown to improve or lower the risk of heart disease and therefore death, and so it's important that you follow your doctor's advice in treating your high cholesterol.

My message here is that if you treat one sign, such as high cholesterol, and don't address all the other health issues, you can be left with a crappy life.

What About The Side Effects Of Cholesterol Drugs?

Cholesterol-lowering drugs have been proven to reduce the number of deaths from cardiovascular disease. Like most drugs, they have also been shown to produce side effects. I find that there are a lot of people who are scared of the cholesterol medications. These medicines seem to have received quite a bit of bad press. It is not unusual for people coming in to my pharmacy to ask me if there is some safe and natural alternative to their prescription medicine. Of all the medicines that we dispense currently, the one that does seem to cause the most concern for people is one group of cholesterol-lowering medications called the "statins." Their common names are simvastatin and atorvastatin. These medications block an enzyme called HMG-CoA reductase, which is the enzyme that is responsible for making cholesterol in your body.

Where Does Cholesterol Come From

I should point out that you make 70% of your cholesterol in your body and you only get 30% of that from your diet on average. That is the general split, but it does differ in different people. So by blocking that enzyme, you block the production of 70% of your cholesterol, so your cholesterol levels decrease.

Downstream Problems From Blocking Cholesterol

Cast your mind back to the picture of the problem of the water running through the paddock in an earlier chapter. By completely blocking the water up-stream the problem seems to be fixed, but the water will likely build up and spill out somewhere else. Well downstream problems are one of the main concerns with the statin cholesterol medicines. Following our example, if you block the water running through the paddock, you might lower the levels of a lower pond, which may remove the water supply for the farm animals.

Getting back to cholesterol medicines, by powerfully blocking an enzyme involved in cholesterol production you also block the production of another important substance in your body called Coenzyme Q10. So the statin medicines lower cholesterol levels, but also your Coenzyme Q10 levels.

The Importance Of CoEnzyme Q10

Coenzyme Q10 is vitally important for energy production in the body. So the first thing we see with someone getting side effects from a statin medicine is a lot of tiredness. If that is not addressed and not treated it can progress to muscle soreness. And in fact, if it goes on unchecked, it can produce a medical condition called rhabdomyolysis, which is extreme muscle breakdown and that's an emergency situation.

Warning Signs That You Need To Watch For

So the key message here is to be alert for any unexplained tiredness or muscle soreness or even cramps. If you have these symptoms, then you need to talk to your doctor and discuss these symptoms and put in place a treatment plan. This plan may involve changing your medication, or supplementing with the nutrients that are depleted by that medication, or both. It is important that you come up with options to give you protection from cardiovascular disease and maintain your quality of life, by avoiding the side effects of tiredness and muscle aches and pains. For this reason, make sure that your health practitioner has an awareness of both conventional and complementary medicines, so you can achieve the best of both worlds.

What Other Nutrients Should I Take If I'm Taking Cholesterol Medication?

In the last chapter we referred to the likely depletion of coenzyme Q10 levels with the continued use of statin medicines. That's the obvious nutrient to consider when taking medicines to lower your cholesterol levels. I get some really great reports from my patients that start taking it. A lot of people think that being tired is quite normal for someone of their age or someone as busy as them. But once they understand the relationship between their medicine and coenzyme Q10 and start taking a supplement of coenzyme Q10, they often come back with something like, "Wow, that's like a turbo boost to my energy levels. I didn't realize how tired I was."

So they get a really big boost in energy which has a dramatic affect on their enjoyment of life. I just love hearing such success stories from my patients. While regaining their boundless energy is the most common feedback we get, coenzyme Q10 is also important for heart health. Coenzyme Q10 lowers blood pressure, improves kidney function, improves eye problems such as age-related macular degeneration, is useful to assist with a healthy immune system, and has even found use with athletes to enhance their performance. There are a whole lot of things in the body that coenzyme Q10 is useful for, not just energy production, so it's really important to maintain good levels of coenzyme Q10.

Treat The Cause

We have mentioned the importance of treating the actual cause of the high cholesterol, which in itself is not a disease. It's just a risk factor for getting heart disease or a stroke. So if you want to prevent heart disease, there are number of nutrients that are important.

Health From Fish

Fish oils have been shown to reduce death from heart attack by 50%. I don't know of any prescription medicine that can claim to have such powerful effects. So eating four meals of oily fish a week or taking a therapeutic dose of a good fish oil supplement can reduce your risk of dying from cardiovascular disease.

The Magic Of Magnesium

Magnesium is an important mineral that reduces heart disease which is the goal in treating high cholesterol. Magnesium in itself can actually control your cholesterol. Magnesium has effects on the same enzyme that the statin medicines work on, namely HMGCoA reductase. However, instead of blocking this enzyme like the statin medicines do, magnesium acts as a moderator of the enzyme. In moderating the action of this enzyme it is not as strong as the statin medicines are, but it is a lot more responsive to what the body needs. For example, if you've got too much cholesterol being produced, magnesium will slow the enzyme down. However, if you have insufficient cholesterol being produced for the body's needs, then magnesium will speed up the enzyme. So it's more like a gate on the river rather than the big boulder that we talked about in the beginning, which allows your body to adjust to its day-to-day requirements.

Obviously if you've got very high cholesterol levels then magnesium is probably not going to be strong enough to bring your levels back down. What is interesting is that magnesium is important for energy production in the body. If you have any signs of cramp in the body or muscle twitches, which are physical signs of magnesium deficiency, then you need to boost your magnesium levels up. Magnesium is involved in over 300 different enzyme processes in the body so if you see early signs of deficiency, you need to correct those because it will affect your health at some stage and possibly in a serious way. There is a summary table of the key signs and symptoms of magnesium deficiency in a later chapter.

Vitamin B3

Vitamin B3 has been shown to be really good for improving cholesterol levels. It has been shown to increase your good cholesterol and lower your bad cholesterol, as well as lowering your triglycerides. Improving your level of triglycerides is important for cardiovascular health but is an area that conventional medication struggled to do successfully.

I need to give a word of caution regarding the doses of vitamin B3. For improvement of cholesterol levels you need to take vitamin B3 in very high doses. These are not the doses you can get from your diet. In fact, the dosage is about 100 times the recommended daily allowance of vitamin B3. I guess you could say that you need to use vitamin B3 like a drug rather than a vitamin based on the dosages required. And because you use it in high levels, you need to take care to use the well tolerated form that does not cause flushing or liver toxicity problems.

Controlling Inflammation

Inflammation is the key cause of heart disease, so trying to find the cause of inflammation and treating the cause will go a long way to improving your heart health. In addition to testing your blood pressure and your cholesterol, doctors are now testing patients for C-reactive protein (CRP). CRP is a marker of inflammation in your body, which they now realize is one of the main predictors of heart disease. So it is now quite widely believed that heart disease is an inflammatory disease.

Identifying the causes of inflammation is a very labour intensive process. The causes are different in different people. I have certainly identified and corrected mine, so it can be done. However, because it does take a lot of time to identify causes of inflammation, conventional doctors don't do very well in this area.

Don't Forget Digestion

If you remember from previous chapters, we discussed how the gastrointestinal system was very important to the immune system and the control of inflammation. So once again we come back to the importance of digestive function in overall health and in this case cardiovascular health.

Now digestive problems won't be the cause of heart disease for everyone. But the key message I would like you to understand is that if you are serious about preventing the number one killer disease for New Zealanders, then you must work with a health practitioner that has a good understanding of all the possible causes of heart disease and will spend the time understanding what is going on in your body.

So What Else Can I Do To Improve My Heart Function?

We all want to live a long life and everyone has different goals about what they want to do with their life. When I ask my patients what their goals are, a lot respond that they want to see their grand kids grow up and marry. That is a great goal for providing long term motivation to start to get fit and to stay healthy well into your old age. The importance of these goals cannot be over-emphasised.

Get Good Advice To Save Wasting Your Money

We have mentioned the importance of fish oils and magnesium. Just a word of caution here, the dosage of your fish oil, and the quality of your magnesium supplements are important.

Magnesium is a big mineral and so the formulation that is used in supplements is vitally important to ensure that what you put into your mouth actually gets into your cells. This is the concept of false economy. There is no point in saving a few dollars when buying your magnesium supplement if you are buying a poorly absorbed form. I have learned this the hard way in my clinic.

In the early days, when patients used to ask me if they could use cheaper products, I would advise them to give it a try. But I found over time, we often could not get the results with a cheaper product. Most of these patients eventually switched to a better brand and got the results they we were seeking. But this ended up costing them more in the long run.

High Cholesterol Is Heart Disease

When I talk to patients in my pharmacy who are getting medicines for blood pressure or cholesterol, many do not realize that they have heart disease. It is not uncommon for one of my pharmacy patients who are taking medications for high blood pressure and cholesterol to say "I just have a little bit of blood pressure, I don't have heart disease." While I don't want to alarm anyone, it is important to realize that if blood pressure is raised, then something is not right in your cardiovascular system. You are at increased risk of heart disease, which is why your doctor has prescribed you blood pressure-lowering medicines. Blood pressure medications are not a vaccination to prevent heart disease, they are a treatment for existing heart disease!

High blood pressure could be due to a number of factors including lifestyle factors such as stress, or nutrient factors such as low levels of magnesium. Magnesium has been shown to lower blood pressure in patients who are deficient.

Fight For Your Health

As you know, I am a pharmacist in a pharmacy and a nutrition medicine practitioner in a nutrition medicine clinic. Comparing the two groups of patients is quite interesting. The patients who come to my clinic are mostly a lot sicker than the patients that enter my pharmacy. They are also less likely to accept that feeling unwell is just part of life. And that is why they have been to multiple doctors, specialists, alternative health practitioners and are now looking to me for their health solutions.

Having such sick people relying on you for help can be daunting. But through the tools of nutrition medicine, most of these people achieve health and vitality again. It can also be inspiring working with these people who are real fighters.

Maybe it's because most of the patients that I see in my pharmacy are not as sick as my clinic patients, but my pharmacy customers seem to be more accepting of poor health. For example, I was chatting with a pharmacy customer recently about how he was going with his prescription medicines. I always like to ask if there are any problems they are having with their medicines. I got the usual "no problems at all" answer. People seem to treat such questions as they would the standard "how are you?" greeting. That is, they just say "fine thanks" even if they are not, since most people assume no-one really wants to know how you are feeling. But of course I genuinely do care about how my customers are feeling. So knowing the most likely side effects of his medications I enquired about some specific problems, namely tiredness and energy levels.

His belief was that feeling tired all day and not being able to do any physically demanding activities was just a normal consequence of getting older. In fact, his response to my specific questions was "No more tired than usual. I have to have a nap twice a day, and I can't mow the lawns anymore. But I am 71 years old now."

I Don't Know What Feeling Good Feels Like

I have to admit it is quite common to become less energetic as we get older, but that is because some metabolic pathway in the body is not working properly. Often that is the result of nutrient deficiencies, which can arise from taking medications.

By now I had a few alarm bells ringing in my brain. So I asked about some key signs of magnesium deficiency. Within five minutes I had a pretty good idea that this man was deficient in magnesium. He was grateful that I had taken the time to take an interest in his health. He was also glad he listened, since he came back a week later saying he felt like he had a lot more energy. Still not 100%, but well on the way to being able to enjoy his life more.

Helping people like this man is a great feeling. Not only in knowing that he feels more vibrant, but knowing that I potentially could have saved a fatal arrhythmia or heart attack or many other potential outcomes associated with low levels of magnesium is a pretty good feeling.

Resveratrol: The New Kid On The Block

Resveratrol is another interesting nutrient for heart disease. A lot of people know that a glass of red wine a day protects their heart. Research indicates that the nutrient in red wine which protects the heart is resveratrol. Resveratrol has been shown to improve heart function, reduce oxidative stress and improve well-being.

I guess any discussion about what you should do to ensure heart health would not be complete without mentioning co-enzyme Q10. We have previously discussed how cholesterol-lowering medications can interfere with co-enzyme Q10 levels and how this can affect energy levels and muscle pain. What you may not be aware of is that co-enzyme Q10 has direct effects on the cardiovascular system. Possible benefits of co-enzyme Q10 include:

- stabilising the heart beat in arrhythmias,
- reducing the hardening of arteries by preventing the oxidation of cholesterol,
- lowering blood pressure,
- preventing stroke.

Coenzyme Q10 Saves Two Legs

One story that left me convinced about the benefits of co-enzyme Q10 did not actually come from one of my patients, but from a presentation that I went to by a cardiologist. Just to give you the highlights, this cardiologist was skeptical about the benefits of co-enzyme Q10 until he worked with a patient who had very poor circulation. This patient was scheduled for surgery to amputate both his legs. A colleague of his convinced him to try treating him with co-enzyme Q10 while they were waiting for the surgery date. There were enough improvements by the date of surgery that they postponed the amputation. Six months later this man was able to walk around a golf course with the use of his own legs. Pretty powerful stuff! I should point out that the doses of co-enzyme Q10 used in this patient were about 6-times higher than we normally use in our pharmacy.

The Evidence Is Strong

By now you are probably thinking that this guy loves his supplements. The reason I have mentioned a few of the supplements that are useful in treating and preventing heart disease is that there is lots of research proving their effectiveness. However, from my clinical experience the most important thing you can do to prevent heart disease is ensure a good diet. In fact, no-one disputes the importance of diet in preventing heart disease. However, knowing what makes up a healthy diet, and then sticking to that diet is the hardest work of all.

To be honest, some people would rather "pop a pill" than have to change their diet. I see that a lot with people who come in to the pharmacy to lose weight. Despite knowing that diet changes are healthier and have a much greater chance of long term success, many patients choose to pop a pill instead. As an aside, one of the most popular weight loss pills has recently been withdrawn from the market because of the increased risk of serious side effects such as stroke and heart attack. Unfortunately, sometimes the easy option is not always the best option.

The Poly-Pill Versus The Poly-Meal

The concept of the poly-pill, which is combining five different medicines into one "pill," has recently been researched. One clever nutrition specialist has copied this approach and come up with the idea of a Poly-meal. They identify six foods that when taken will reduce the risk of a heart attack or stroke by over 70%. Wow that is a huge reduction in risk! In other words, instead of taking five tablets, you just make sure you've got the six key foods in your diet.

The Polymeal Approach To Preventing Heart Disease: every day consume:

- One glass of red wine (150ml)
- Dark chocolate (100g) (should NOT contain dairy products)
- Almonds (68g)
- Garlic (2.7g)
- Fruit and vegetables (400g)

Plus consume fish (118g of oily fish preferably) at least four times a week.

Recently a lady came to see me because her cholesterol levels, while not overly high, were heading towards the high-risk category. Her doctor had said that if her cholesterol didn't improve she would need to start taking medicines. She wanted to be around long enough to see her grandkids go off to school, so she was quite motivated. However, she was reluctant to start taking cholesterol medications. She agreed to change her diet, incorporating the principles of the polymeal.

When she came back after her next doctors visit, she was pleased that her cholesterol levels had improved slightly, but she was even more delighted that she felt so much better. She felt healthy and she had lost a bit of weight as well. All this was achieved solely with changing the diet.

So that's a really encouraging story for us; not only did that lady get all the benefits from reduced heart attack risk and has the ability to achieve her life goals, but she just feels so much better today and she does not have to worry about any medication side effects.

7

Antibiotics

Overuse

There is a common belief amongst the medical profession that antibiotics are overused. The medical profession has worked pretty hard to try and reduce the amount of antibiotics that are used.

Back about 30 years ago, antibiotics were sometimes prescribed for patients that had any sort of sniffle or fever, whether serious or trivial and whether or not it was caused by a bacteria. This has lead to the development of bacteria that are resistant to antibiotics, the so called super bugs.

So now there is a common belief among medical authorities that the use of antibiotics should be limited to cases where their use is absolutely necessary.

Underuse

Some patients I talk to think that antibiotics are evil and should be avoided at all costs. However, antibiotics are a very important class of medications and they should be used when required for the right indication at the right time and in the right dose.

If you need an antibiotic, you should not be afraid to use one. Many advances in health have come from reducing the impact of infectious diseases by using antibiotics and also by improving hygiene standards to reduce the rate of infection. I actually encourage some of my patients to go to their doctor and get prescriptions for antibiotics when I know they have a bacterial infection or overgrowth that will not respond to diet and nutrient interventions.

A Real Life Example

To illustrate this point let me tell you about a patient who recently came to see me after being ill for a very long time. Her main complaints were frequent nausea and diarrhoea, a lack of energy, inability to sleep and lately she had been having trouble concentrating. All the tests that the doctors had ordered for her were normal. On questioning her about various phases of her life, it became apparent that she had suffered from severe allergic diseases when she was younger and had received a lot of antibiotics for various infections.

My first thoughts for this patient was that she had allergic or sensitivity reactions to a number of foods, which had caused inflammation in the gut. This inflammation plus the history of regular antibiotic use made me suspect an imbalance in the gut, especially involving the good and bad bacteria in the gut.

We changed her diet and she had an immediate improvement in symptoms. We put her on a number of supplements to boost energy production and she found she could swim a lot further than normal.

However, after about three months her stomach bloating and diarrhoea began to return. So we did some extra tests on her and found that she had an overgrowth of bad bacteria in her small intestines. These bacteria were shown to produce a lot of hydrogen gas (hence the bloating). Now because these bad bacteria were well established and hadn't disappeared when we improved the diet, we had to resort to using antibiotics to kill them off.

So I wrote a referral to her doctor, who wrote a prescription for the right antibiotics for those particular bacteria. For this patient we needed to use a small steady dose over an extended period of time. Simultaneously, we used high doses of a specific probiotic (the good bacteria), so that they would colonise the gastrointestinal tract and prevent the wrong bacteria from coming back. Her health improved again and at last report she had not had any further symptoms.

The reason I highlight this case is to show that antibiotics are not bad. They are an essential tool that has been somewhat overused. But if reserved for appropriate cases and if supplemented with probiotics, then they can be beneficial for patients.

When Not To Use An Antibiotic

While acknowledging the importance of antibiotics in some instances, we still see patients who are prescribed antibiotics for what is most likely to be a viral infection. Antibiotics by definition are medicines that kill bacteria, not viruses. The best defence against viruses is a strong immune system. This is because viruses mutate (change their characteristics) regularly so it is difficult to design a medicine that will be effective against them. Your own immune system on the other hand, is good at changing with the viruses, and if healthy can stay one step ahead of viruses.

We also still see antibiotics prescribed for conditions like glue ear despite the fact that studies indicate there is no advantage and no benefit in the use of antibiotics for patients with glue ear. In fact, given the potential to disrupt the good bacteria in the gut, the overall risks outweigh the benefits.

A Tragic Story

Ensuring the appropriate use of antibiotics is a responsibility that we all have. Not just doctors, but patients sometimes put doctors under pressure to prescribe antibiotics for them when they clearly are not needed. I feel very strongly about this. Let me tell you why. When I was at university, one of my friends died from septicemia, which is an overgrowth of bacteria in the blood. Perhaps if she had received antibiotics sooner, or if there was less bacterial resistance to antibiotics then she might still be alive today.

Complementing Your Medicine With A Probiotic?

If you do need to take an antibiotic, then you should take it as advised by your pharmacist. If you have a good pharmacist, then he or she will describe how many to take, how often to take them, the timing of the dosages with respect to food, whether or not you need to complete the course, and what you need to do to ensure the best outcomes from this antibiotic. This will normally involve taking a probiotic (the good bacteria) to replace the good bacteria that may be killed off by the antibiotic.

Listening Could Save Your Life

It pays to listen to your pharmacist's advice. If you fly on a plane from time to time, you will be familiar with the safety briefing from the aircrew: "should an oxygen mask appear in front of you...." If you have heard this message regularly, it is quite easy to dismiss it. But your life depends on it.

We occasionally get people in our pharmacy who don't seem to want to listen to our advice about how to get the best health from their medicines. When we start to assume we know what to do, that is when mistakes happen.

A few years ago, my wife Christine needed a course of antibiotics. The doctor prescribed doxycycline 100mg one tablet each day for five days. Now I assumed that since Christine is a smart lady, she would read the label thoroughly and take the right dosage, so I didn't bother to give her the usual level of counseling that one of my patients would get.

After just one day, she said to me that she was going to need some more tablets, since she had just about used them all up. So

I replied that it was only supposed to be a short five day course and she wouldn't need any more after that. Christine then said that there wasn't even enough for two days. "How many are you taking," I asked. "The usual ... one tablet three times a day," she replied. She was supposed to be taking only one a day, not three. Luckily no harm was done in this case. However, medicines are very powerful substances and we need to be extra careful and not get blasé about their use.

The Good And The Bad

Having a balance of the right bacteria in the gastrointestinal tract is one of the most important factors in ensuring good health. Good bacteria are always in a constant battle with bad bacteria and any pathogens entering the body, so you need a good healthy set of gut bacteria.

As we mentioned earlier, 70% or more of your immune system resides in the gut, and a good healthy mix of gut bacteria will help to keep your immune system in tip top shape. The good bacteria are one of your first defenses against invaders coming into the body.

So my recommendation is that if you are a healthy person and you have been prescribed a short course of antibiotics to ward off a mild infection, then take a probiotic for the duration of the antibiotic course plus a week afterwards. That should be enough just to maintain that normal healthy level that you had before you took your antibiotic.

On the other hand, if you have a history of illness before your course of antibiotics, then you might be best to take a prolonged course of a probiotic. Remember my clinic patient that needed a long-term course of antibiotics? Obviously we needed a long-term course of probiotics to go with that. In fact, we had to use a special probiotic for her based on the balance of the bacteria that were in her gut. Luckily we had done this test and knew exactly which good bacteria she was going to need.

Inconvenient Side Effects Of Antibiotics

We do have some patients in the pharmacy that ask if they really need a probiotic since they didn't get any diarrhoea last time they took an antibiotic. What they need to understand is that there are short term side effects of antibiotics such as thrush for women and diarrhea for men and women. Some people will get those and some people won't. And so if you didn't get thrush or diarrhoea last time, that's great. You might not again. It depends on the antibiotic too, as some are stronger than others in terms of killing off those gut bacteria.

Serious Side Effects Of Antibiotics

The more significant adverse effects of antibiotics are the long term effects on health. You may not notice these effects straight away, but they can dramatically affect your health. In fact, one of the standard questions I ask in my clinic practice is how often you have had antibiotics in the past. This is important as it alerts me to the possibility of an imbalance in gut bacteria as a cause of gut inflammation and subsequent poor health. I should point out that it is quite common for these chronically ill patients to have taken frequent courses of antibiotics early in their life. It appears that antibiotic use in the first two years of life puts patients at higher risk of health problems later in life.

We have previously discussed the role of inflammation in seemingly unrelated diseases like heart disease. By now you are hopefully getting an understanding of the importance of gut health, which includes the balance of good and bad bacteria, in the immune system and inflammation. Perhaps less known adverse consequences of upsetting the balance of the good and bad bacteria include:

- reduced efficiency of the immune system, meaning you are more likely to get sick again;
- inflammation in the gastrointestinal tract making you

more susceptible to allergies;
- impaired absorption of nutrients which can result in many of your metabolic pathways not working properly;
- impaired brain function. The gut is a complex interaction of nerves and is sometimes referred to as the "second brain."

An Imbalance Of Bacteria Can Contribute To Devastating Disease

So you can see that almost any disease can come about from an imbalance of the good and bad bacteria. To illustrate this, let me tell you about a young woman who came to see me about her autistic child. This child appeared quite normal until the age of two, then went downhill fast. His behavior was so bad that the family could not take him out of the house. His mum could not leave the house either. This child's illness was not only devastating his life, but also his family's happiness.

I recommended that this woman take her son to see a doctor that specializes in treating autistic children through nutrition medicine. There is quite a lot of evidence that for some patients with autism, there is an imbalance in the metabolism of metals and severe intolerance of some foods. So with the help of this specialist we worked on this child's zinc-dependent enzymes, but also on his digestion, including correcting the balance of good and bad bacteria. Now this is one of my happiest stories. This child gradually improved under this rigorous treatment protocol and by the age of five was able to go to a normal school. He remained a little behind his peers in terms of his intellectual development, but at least he was well enough to go to school. The relief for this boy's family was immense as you can imagine.

From my clinic practice I see the sometimes dramatic effects on health of an imbalance of gut bacteria. So I guess I can be forgiven if I get a little intense about the need for probiotics with antibiotics. I certainly would not take an antibiotic or let anyone in my family take one without taking a probiotic during and afterwards. And since I do truly care about my customers in my pharmacy, I make sure they understand why they need take a probiotic when they take an antibiotic.

Should I Take My Probiotic During The Course Of Antibiotics Or After?

By now I hope I have enlightened you on why you need to take a probiotic with an antibiotic. The next question is then how do you take it to get the best effects. The jury is still out on whether you should start your probiotic at the same time as your antibiotic or whether you should start taking it once you have finished the antibiotic. We do know from studies of taking medicines that clear out the bowel (eg. before surgery), that the bowel will recolonise with new bacteria very quickly, usually within 24 hours. So you can't leave it a long time before you start your probiotics.

On the other hand if you take your probiotic at the same time as your antibiotics, you may get a reasonable number of them killed off. On balance, I like to recommend my patients start taking their probiotic on the same day they start taking their antibiotic, but at a different time of the day. Plus, I recommend taking a probiotic for at least an extra week after you have finished the antibiotic. For example, if you have been prescribed an antibiotic for one week, I'd say take your probiotic during that week and for at least another week, if you're healthy. For patients with a history of illness, I will get them to take it for a longer period of time.

Some recent research I was reading recently suggested that a probiotic should be part of the normal supplements every day. Certainly, they need to be taken not at the same time of the day as the antibiotic, but a couple of hours apart. That helps them to avoid being killed off too early. They need to be kept in the fridge where they maintain most of their potency.

Quality Counts With Probiotics

The other important thing about probiotics is the quality of the brand. This includes the purity of the product, the type and number of bacteria which contribute to the effectiveness, and the presence of possible excipients. For example, if the good bacteria in your probiotic is grown on media that contains dairy and you have a dairy sensitivity, then that's going to disrupt your gut function and counteract what you're trying to do. So in our pharmacy we have for our patients different species of bacteria depending on the needs of their gut and depending on any sort of dietary issues or food sensitivities that they may have.

How Do We Tell A Good Quality Probiotic From A Bad?

It's not easy to know which supplements are good quality when you're a consumer. You can be bombarded with advertising material, they often look similar and contain really large names like bifidobacteria or lactobacillus. So it can be hard to know which is best. But if you talk to your pharmacist about which one is right for you, they should have an understanding of which good bacteria are important for which particular health issues that you might have. For example, if you have an acute episode of diarrhoea, you will want to take a high dose of a strong probiotic. Whereas for replacing the good bacteria in an otherwise healthy person after an antibiotic, a standard combination of lactobacillus and bifidobacteria is a good way to start. But you need to talk to your pharmacist in case you have other issues that need to be taken into account.

So How Do You Know Which Probiotic Is The Best One For You?

You really need some expert guidance on that. It is not an area that gets covered very well at Pharmacy school. But some pharmacists have done extra training. They have been to extra courses and have the skills to know which good bacteria are important in which situations.

In my clinic, when I am faced with a very sick person I prefer to test what bacteria are actually present in the gut before deciding which probiotic I will use. I had a patient in this week and I ended up using three different products to get the coverage she needed based on her test results.

But for most patients that I see in my pharmacy, we can choose the strain of bacteria that is most appropriate for their symptoms. For example, Lactobacillus rhamnosis is a strain of bacteria that tends to work well in patients with eczema. Lactobacillius plantarum on the other hand tends to work well for people with irritable bowel syndrome. However, if you are otherwise healthy, and just need to complement your antibiotic prescription, then a mix of Lactobacillus and Bifidobacteria is a good multi-purpose option.

Are There Any Side Effects From Probiotics?

Probiotics are pretty safe. When you think about it, you are really only putting into your body what should be there to start with. Some brands have extra nutrients and additives which can cause problems. For example one brand that we stock contains several of the B vitamins as well as vitamin K. These extra nutrients are important, since they are depleted when the antibiotics kill off the good bacteria. So again, they are replacing what your body would normally produce. However, patients may be sensitive to these extra vitamins. If you are on strong blood thinning medications like warfarin and the doctor prescribes antibiotics, you can expect to be more sensitive to warfarin. Taking probiotics, especially those that contain vitamin K, will help to prevent this. Vitamin K has a direct effect on the medication warfarin.

Another fairly common additive in probiotics is fructooligosaccharide (FOS). Normally, it helps the good bacteria grow by providing the food source for them. However, I have a few patients in my clinic who have reacted to probiotics containing FOS that they have received from other practitioners. I suspect that these patients have a fructose intolerance.

The probiotic bacteria themselves are pretty well tolerated. Occasionally, certain strains can cause problems for people that are a little bit sensitive. For example, a couple of the main strains of bacteria produce acid in the colon and intestines where they have their effect. This can create problems in terms of interfering with digestion at that level of the gut. If you want to be sure, you need to get a nutrition medicine pharmacist to talk to you about these issues. It's quite a detailed complex area and most pharmacists probably won't have the training or clinical experience in this area. If you're going to use probiotics in the long term, or if you are elderly, then you need to really get expert advice on what species of good bacteria are right for you, so you achieve the best of health and avoid any imbalances in the mix of bacteria in the gut.

My Son's Story

I actually put my youngest son on probiotics for three years when he was three years old. He was starting to get quite regular respiratory infections. His immune system seemed to be quite impaired. In fact, he had been to the doctor for infections about six times in the previous six months. We put him on a probiotic and we kept him on that until he was six years old. The ages of three through to six are quite a high risk time for kids to pick up bugs, since they start attending daycare centres and school. But in that three-year period he didn't need to go to the doctor at all. So he had a really impressive response to the probiotics and had no side effects from taking it for that long. It really seems to have given his immune system a huge boost.

8

Anti-Depressants And
Sleeping Pills

Do I Really Have Depression?

With nutrition medicine, we believe in the concept of biochemical individuality, which means everyone is different. So it's a bit hard to say whether an antidepressant is appropriate or not. For some people the antidepressant medications are appropriate and are very helpful in getting people through a tough patch.

However, there is now a push in conventional medicine to utilize counseling and other forms of psychotherapy as a preference to the antidepressant medications. This is because of the effectiveness and safety concerns about the medications.

Inappropriate Use

We often see patients who have chronic conditions like chronic fatigue, fibromyalgia or irritable bowel syndrome, which tends to be difficult to treat with conventional medicines. You can understand that a caring doctor does want to help these patients. But since they do not have any tools in their toolkit that will make a difference, they reach for an antidepressant. Often these patients will get depressed about their condition, and at least the antidepressants make them feel a bit better about themselves, even though the underlying condition has not been addressed.

So for people with such a chronic condition, I'd say an antidepressant isn't indicated and they need to address the causes of their ill health and then their mood and happiness with their life will improve subsequent to that.

First Do No Harm

The primary guiding principle taught to medical professionals is to first do no harm. Anti-depressants do have side effects, so using them in conditions that they are not indicated for is potentially putting a patient at risk unnecessarily. It comes back to balancing the benefits versus the risks for individual patients.

Major depressive disorders do need to be treated because they can be life threatening based on the increased risk of suicides. Plus people just can't function when their depression gets severe. With more minor levels of depression, it's really up to the patient themselves to decide how much it is interfering with their quality of life and their ability to function. They may be able to make a decision to work through their depression with behavioural techniques, counseling, the support of their family and friends and even a walk along the beach or walk in the bush which can help to clear your mind and improve your outlook on life.

A Debilitated Lady

One of my first patients, let's call her Karen, came to me having a 20-year history of depression starting at age 14. Now, it was assumed her problems were hormonally related because they co-incided with the onset of puberty. She came to me because I had done a lot of work with patients balancing their hormones and I had a lot of success with those patients. In the process of my consultation with her, I discovered that at the age of 14, her dentist had put fillings in all of her teeth just to prevent her getting any decay in her teeth. So my mind obviously started thinking about the possibility of heavy metal toxicity. Mercury is very damaging to nerves if it leaches out of fillings.

Over the subsequent 20 years, she had been prescribed a range of anti-depressants, which helped her to function. She mentioned to me that she never felt really well, and had gone through those last 20 years in "a bit of a fog." As part of my nutrition medicine assessment, I analysed her diet and performed a few tests. I discovered that she had digestive problems, had low intake of protein and her hormones were unbalanced such that she was breaking down lean tissue rather than building it up. The combination of these factors meant that she had a very low availability of protein in the body. This was significant because protein contains amino acids which are the building blocks of the brain chemicals.

So we changed her diet, prescribed a few supplements for her and added some complementary therapies. We got her to a stage where she was feeling really good. Then in consultation with her doctor, they agreed to try and reduce the dose of her medication. She eventually was able to discontinue her anti-depressants after 20 years. She could not believe just how good she was feeling. In her words, she was seeing life and experiencing life just so clearly. It was like a whole fog had been lifted. Karen's story illustrates a case where anti-depressant therapy was needed, but maybe a combination of some nutrition medicine options, or an initial trial of some of the natural options with less side effects might have been better for her at the earlier stages.

What Are The Side Effects Of Antidepressants?

Like many categories of medications, there are common effects that you would expect from any antidepressant as well as some additional effects that are specific to individual antidepressants. Many antidepressants will cause some sort of drowsiness and so we often will get around it by getting the patient to take it at nighttime and so they're drowsy at nighttime, which is not a bad thing. However, because these medications can have long lasting effects, patients often complain about being drowsy the next day, or what is commonly referred to as a hangover effect the next day. One of my patients at the moment has been in a real dilemma with his anti-depressant dose. The higher the dose of his medication the more effective it is, but also the more drowsy he gets. So he has been trying to find a balance of a happy functional level without getting too sleepy the next day. Because he is quite sensitive to the side effects of his medication, he has come to me to look at other alternatives that will help to improve his outlook on life and his mood and allow him to reduce the dose of his antidepressant medications.

Hangover effects are a major problem for a lot of patients and is one of the reasons why they don't want to take those medications. They just don't feel energetic and vibrant. Their mood improves on them, but they know that they're not alert and as active as they could be. There are also other side effects like dry mouth. Now a dry mouth doesn't sound so serious, but it actually can be very irritating for patients. In fact, for some people, these irritations can be strong enough that they will decide to stop their medications or seek a different one from their doctor.

Complementing Your Prescription

When dealing with depression there is a need to balance complementary and conventional medications to help patients achieve good health. Conventional medications can't help anyone that refuses to take them because of side effects. So for these patients it is valid to consider alternative treatments, of which there are many.

A Lesson In Biochemisty

A lot of the most popular medications work on serotonin. Serotonin is one of the brain chemicals or neurotransmitters, and low levels of serotonin in the body is associated with low mood and depression. At the risk of getting a bit technical, let me explain how these medicines affect serotonin in the body. These medications stop serotonin being re-absorbed back into the nerve terminal, and so you get more effect from it.

Think of serotonin as like orange juice, your nerve as the orange and the nerve synapse as the glass that holds the juice. The more juice in the glass the better. What the medications do is stop the juice in the glass being recycled back into the orange. So the juice stays in the glass. So using these antidepressants is like squeezing the last bit of juice out of an orange. The problem with this is that after a while you just run out of juice to squeeze out of that same orange.

Running Out Of Juice

Now this reduced amount of juice can have a couple of consequences. First the effects of these medicines tend to reduce in the long term. So that's why we see patients who are on these medicines for long periods of time needing to swap medications or increase the dose.

Secondly, because there is less total orange juice in the body, it is often difficult to stop taking these medications without getting a dramatic worsening of symptoms. This is known as a rebound or withdrawal effect, and patients can feel trapped on their medications.

A better course of action than squeezing the orange to death, is to add more oranges into the system. In other words, it is better to put more serotonin into the nerve terminal or have more serotonin available in the body rather than overuse the last stores of serotonin. It makes sense and people can get a lot better health outcomes that way. Serotonin actually comes from protein, so it is no surprise again that diet (and of course digestion and absorption) can play a big role in how much serotonin we have in our body.

Natural Strategies To Improve Mood

There is a huge range of nutrients that people have used for improving mood. But before considering what nutrients might be best for my patients, I look at the lifestyle or environmental triggers that might be present. Obviously, stress is a major cause of depression. For some of my patients, it is not possible to eliminate the causes of stress, but there are lifestyle strategies that can help to keep stress under control. For example, meditation, yoga, listening to music or exercise can help make stress more manageable.

Exercise can be quite therapeutic as long as it is not too intense. It is better to just begin with a gentle walk along the beach. Speaking of the beach, mood is quite strongly affected by negative ions. Negative ions are really helpful for health, happiness and joy. You get a lot of negative ions coming off the ocean at the beach, so a walk on the beach can be therapeutic. Not just for the exercise but for those negative ions. Similarly, a walk in the bush can increase the negative ions that your body has.

Positive ions work in the opposite way and are detrimental to health. You get positive ions from working under fluorescent lights, around electronic devices and in "toxic buildings." Working by computer screens can give you a big dose of positive ions. Therefore, after your day at work, taking a walk through the park or along the beach on your way to your car and taking deep slow breaths can do wonders for your mood and overall health.

Helpful Supplements

When it comes to actual supplements that you can use, St. John's wort is one herb that has been used a lot by naturopaths and is very effective. It has a down side in that it interferes with some enzymes in the liver. This means that it speeds up these enzymes which reduces the levels of some medicines in the body. So you should be very careful if you're taking a prescription medicine and want to start taking St. John's wort. This includes medicines that you may be using for a completely different condition. It doesn't just include other anti-depressants.

I wouldn't recommend any patient start taking St. John's wort without consulting an experienced pharmacist that knows what they are talking about in terms of drug and nutrient interactions. It could be safe, but you need to find out because the consequences could be quite serious.

We talked about adding more serotonin into the body, or more juice into the oranges. So how do we do this? Serotonin is made from an amino acid called tryptophan, which is one of the amino acids that make up protein. So having more protein in the diet can help increase serotonin levels. A more specific approach is to take more of tryptophan itself, although the metabolite of tryptophan, which is called 5-hydroxytryptamine (5-HTP), appears to be more effective. A lot of the natural anti-depressant supplements will use 5-hydroxytryptamine because it is more effective than tryptophan.

5-HTP And Orange Juice

Because 5-HTP is an amino acid, taking it with protein-rich food can reduce the amount of absorption. So I always recommend my patients take their 5-HTP with a little bit of carbohydrate, like a little bit of orange juice perhaps. It should not be taken with protein. Now this may sound a bit contradictory, since I mentioned how important protein is for health, but it is important to get the most out of your supplement.

This also emphasizes the importance of consulting a pharmacist with expert knowledge in nutrition medicine and prescription medicine, so you get the right advice and you get the best health outcomes.

The B-Vitamins

The B vitamins are important co-factors for many enzymes in the body. A lot of mood disorders can be caused by deficiencies in B vitamins including anxiety, apathy, confusion, right through to depression, and even Alzheimer's disease. A deficiency of the B vitamins has been implicated as causes of those conditions.

Fish Oils

Fish oils are vitally important for brain function. Your brain is a fatty organ, so getting good fats into your brain means that you are going to have better mental function, including mood and concentration. For example, fantastic improvements in learning, concentration and behavior have been shown in kids with ADHD.

However, it is important to get the right combination of the fish oils in the right dose. The essential fatty acid that is important for the brain is docosahexaenoic acid or DHA. Again, talk to your pharmacist about which fish oil product contains the correct balance and dose of the essential fatty acids for brain health.

SAMe: Works Quickly And Works Well

This book is certainly not supposed to be a comprehensive list of alternative therapies. However, I thought it would be interesting to talk about a substance called S-adenosyl methionine or SAMe (pronounced "sammie"). SAMe is a methylation agent, and without getting into the detail of biochemistry, most reactions that occur in the body are methylation reactions. So you would predict that SAMe might help the body to work. What is really interesting about SAMe is how very effective it is in the treatment of depression. There have been studies involving patients with major depression comparing the use of SAMe against conventional medications. In these studies, SAMe has been shown to be at least as effective as conventional medicines.

One of the problems with conventional medications for depression is there can often be a lag phase between when you start to take the tablets and when you start to feel a positive clinical effect. That is quite a danger for patients with major depression because you want the benefits to start quite quickly.

What actually happens in clinical practice is that when starting antidepressant medications, patients can feel worse for a week or two and sometimes for up to six weeks before starting to feel better. But SAMe is a bit different. It seems to have an effect very quickly. Usually within the first week patients notice the benefit.

These are just a few options of what can help to get the best long term health outcome for patients with depression. It is best to work with a competent health practitioner to determine what is the right treatment for you. You should also remember that counseling and psychotherapy have been shown to be very effective treatments for depression.

How Do I Work Out Which Treatment Is Right For Me?

I've hinted previously that the key message is to get some good advice from a health practitioner that does not have a vested interest in any one treatment type. There's a lot of information on the internet. If you Google anti-depressants you will get a whole lot of information. But if you are not thinking clearly this can be bewildering. There are a number of pitfalls, and there are a number of areas where, if you don't quite know what you're doing, then you might not get the best result. So you may chance upon the right remedy for you, but if you don't take it in the right way, then you will not get the desired effects. There may also be complicating factors to take into account that may have caused the depression in the first place. If you don't identify and treat these underlying causes then you will be fighting a losing battle.

Objective Help

Health practitioners are discouraged from treating themselves or members of their family, since it is difficult to be objective about your own health or that of your loved ones. This is especially so if you have problems with depression, because you will often not be thinking straight. A good pharmacist will have a great knowledge of the nutrients and the supplements that may be useful, whether they be herbs or vitamins and minerals. They will also understand what prescription medications you may be taking and they can look at the interactions between those and therefore understand the complete picture for you.

What Can Be Done To Help Me Sleep?

There are a great range of effective natural sleep remedies. There are also very effective medicines that can help you get to sleep. However, the commonly available prescription medicines for sleep are associated with many problems. Therefore, it surprises me that natural remedies are not used more often by doctors.

Sleeping Pills

The main class of pharmaceuticals used for inducing sleep is called the benzodiazepines. The medicines in this category have different characteristics: some have short actions and get you off to sleep quickly, while some have longer actions and can help you stay asleep in the later stages of your sleep. Unfortunately, all these medicines have a major problem in that they are addictive. What this means is that these medicines are fine if you have short-term problem with sleep or an occasional problem with sleep. For example it would be appropriate to use a benzodiazepine if you were going on a plane and wanted to sleep during the flight.

Addiction Is A Very Real Problem

Unfortunately, disturbances in sleep often happen after a major stressful event or because of other long term health issues, such as inability to sleep because of the pain of arthritis. These patients will likely need help to get to sleep for a long period of several months. By that stage you would likely be addicted to these sleeping tablets, which means that as soon as you try to stop taking them, your sleep problems become much worse, plus the withdrawal effect often leaves you feeling irritated and unhappy. You can imagine how disturbing this could be to someone with anxiety or depression, who doesn't feel well to start with.

The Importance Of Diet To Sleep

For some patients, an inability to sleep can be caused by problems in the diet. For example, we previously explained how important adequate protein intake was to get good levels of the amino acid tryptophan. Tryptophan is an important building block to make serotonin, one of the key brain chemicals that helps you to feel good. What I didn't tell you about in the previous paragraphs is how serotonin then gets converted to melatonin, which is your natural sleep hormone. This process requires a number of cofactors such as vitamin B6. So you can see low levels of protein or vitamin B6 could easily affect sleep by reducing the amount of melatonin available. In fact, poor sleep might be a warning sign that you have a nutrient deficiency. Like the warning light on your car dashboard, it should not be ignored, nor should you cover it up, by which I mean you shouldn't take sleeping tablets without addressing the cause of the poor sleep.

In my pharmacy we see many patients bringing in prescriptions for sleeping tablets. I am sure that most of these people are not aware of how addictive these tablets are. People need to be very cautious about going on to sleeping tablets, and your pharmacist should be counseling you about the need for caution and how to lower your risk of becoming dependent on these sleeping pills. A pharmacist with a good understanding of nutrition medicine will also be able to help you identify the cause of your sleep problems. Certainly sleep is very important for the body to heal and for feeling well the next day, but certainly getting addicted to a drug is not fun at all. In fact, addiction can be devastating.

An Example Of Lost Vitality

I was speaking to a patient from my pharmacy about the dangers of taking sleeping pills over a prolonged period of time. Her argument was that being dependent on a medicine was not a problem since there would always be a continual supply available from her doctor. After a further 10 minutes of me gently poking my nose into her background health, it became apparent there was a number of hormone imbalances underlying the poor sleep. Once I explained to her about how imbalances of one hormone can affect the balance of another, she began to understand the importance of her "warning light" (poor sleep) for her overall health. While I did not recommend that we stop her sleeping tablets, I did recommend that she requested her doctor run a few more tests to confirm where the imbalance was coming from. She corrected her hormone imbalance and started to reduce her use of sleeping tablets. The outcome for this patient was significantly increased energy and vitality during the day, and she slowly reduced her sleeping tablet use down to once or twice a month only.

Melatonin

In a previous paragraph I mentioned that melatonin was the natural sleep hormone that your body produces at night to help you sleep. If for some reason your body can't make enough melatonin, you can take extra melatonin. In some countries you can buy melatonin over-the-counter. In New Zealand, it is a prescription medicine. I am not sure of the exact reasons why melatonin is a prescription medicine in NZ, since it is very safe to take. Perhaps it is to ensure people who cannot sleep well see a doctor to rule out any serious causes of poor sleep.

One of my holiday jobs when I was at university was to clean and load planes for Air New Zealand. We didn't interact much with the cabin staff, but those that I did get to know used to rave about how good melatonin was to help normalize sleep patterns from multiple time zones and unusual work shift patterns.

B Vitamins Give You Energy AND Good Sleep

Back to the biochemistry. To convert serotonin to melatonin requires a co-factor, namely vitamin B6. So if you've got a vitamin B6 deficiency, you're going to have a problem sleeping. You don't need to be a rocket scientist to know that fixing a vitamin B6 deficiency is pretty simple.

Most pharmacies will have a range of B vitamin supplements. The hard part is getting a health practitioner who is smart enough to identify the problem for you. Similarly if you have a vitamin B3 deficiency, your body will take all the tryptophan from your diet and use it to make vitamin B3, leaving no tryptophan available for making serotonin and melatonin.

So before putting my patients at risk of getting addicted to a prescription medicine, I recommend some simple tests to identify potential nutrient deficiencies. There are some classic physical signs of deficiency of the B-vitamins, which I have listed in Chapter 11. If your pharmacist has a good knowledge of all these nutrients and their deficiency signs, then they could help you to identify whether a B-vitamin deficiency might be the cause of your poor sleep. Mostly, you don't need to carry out expensive and uncomfortable blood tests, you can get a good idea of nutrient status from some physical signs and symptoms. For example, signs of a vitamin B6 deficiency include, in addition to poor sleep, not remembering your dreams, a cherry tip on the tongue, seborrhea (oily or shiny skin), and poor wound healing. Signs of vitamin B3 deficiency include bad breath, strawberry tip of the tongue, scalloping and crevassing on the edge of the tongue, and cracks in the corner of the mouth. If you have all these physical signs, then it would be appropriate to try a course of a vitamin B complex.

Take Time To Watch The Sun Go Down

Anyway, back to melatonin the natural sleep hormone. Melatonin is actually made in the pineal glands by the action of the special wavelengths of light at sunset. So if you have the luxury of being able to watch the sun going down in the evening somewhere where it is nice and sunny and you have the time, it's a great way to stimulate your melatonin production.

TV And Computers Disrupt Sleep

What a lot of people don't realize is that blue light will actually interfere with melatonin production. The significance of this is that television produces high levels of blue light. To see for yourself, turn on your television after dark and turn all the lights off. Stand outside the room and observe the colour of the room changing under the influence of the light produced by the television. You will likely be surprised at how much blue light comes from your television room.

Now many people will watch television right up until bedtime, which will interfere with their melatonin production. After a few hours of television (or "anti-sleep" treatment) they go to bed and not surprisingly they can't sleep. Television can keep you awake, not just because the programs are so exciting or they give you bad dreams, but that blue light in pharmacological levels affects melatonin production.

This reminds me of a very straight forward case of insomnia that I helped a patient with. He had a lot of sleep problems and, like a lot of people who start taking prescription medicines for sleep, he was concerned about getting addicted to his sleeping pills and wanted to try alternatives to his sleeping tablets. We certainly got him to turn off his TV after the news had finished at 7pm. We started him on some relaxation exercises, tidied up his diet and started him on a vitamin B complex. It wasn't as easy for him as I'm making it sound, but he did respond very well and slept well without the need for sleeping tablets. He also commented that with less television time, he ended up talking to his family a lot more instead.

9

Asthma

Why Is Asthma So Common Now?

While no-one knows why asthma is more common now, it is a fact that there are a lot more people with asthma now than there used to be. There are many theories that have been put forward.

For example, the hygiene hypothesis states that our obsession with hygiene reduces the exposure of babies and infants to germs and so our immune systems do not develop properly. Another theory suggests that environmental toxins have poisoned our world which damages our immune system.

Allergy As A Cause

Research has demonstrated that many cases of asthma are caused by problems with the immune system and these are usually associated with other illnesses. For example, it is very common for someone with asthma to have irritable bowel syndrome, hay fever or eczema. In my clinic I see a lot of people with eczema in association with asthma. In these people, there is almost always an allergic cause of their condition. What this means is that their immune system reacts to substances, which then cause inflammation throughout the body.

Often these substances that they react to are everyday substances that are difficult to avoid, like foods and air-bourne substances such as pollens and animal dander. But the good news is that when you do identify and remove the causative agent, then the disease condition improves dramatically and many of my patients get complete resolution of symptoms.

Diet

So why would this be more common now than in the past? If we consider the average modern diet, it contains a high level of pesticides, flavourings, colourings and preservatives. This supports the environmental toxin theory. However, modern diets tend to be very high in sugars, which are very inflammatory. When I talk about sugars to patients in my pharmacy, many of them say that they don't eat much sugar at all. However, sugar in the diet is not always obvious. For example, high sugar foods include many cereals, convenience foods (e.g. instant noodles), potatoes, soft drinks, fruit juices, white rice and breads and bakery products. In fact, many sauces are also high in sugar. Hidden sugars are everywhere.

In the United Kingdom, 2.3 billion tons of sugar go into the food supply each year. That is 38 kg of sugar per person per year. If you think that is frightening then what do you think the Americans consume? Well in 1975, Americans consumed a whopping 56 kg of sugar per person. As if this wasn't bad enough, now they consume 71 kg of sugar per person per year! Unfortunately (or maybe fortunately) I don't have the statistics for New Zealand.

I was having a nice tall gin and tonic on my holiday recently. I thought this would be a lot better for me on the hot sunny day than a beer, which is high in sugar and contains gluten. I started to read the label on the tonic water bottle and discovered that tonic water has almost as much sugar as normal soft drinks like cola and lemonade. Sugar, it seems, is everywhere!

Digestion

Anyway, back to the effects of sugar on asthma. A diet that is high in simple sugars can disrupt the gastrointestinal system and cause inflammation throughout the body. Now for someone with asthma in their family, this could be enough to turn on their asthma. Furthermore, once the gastrointestinal system is disrupted, patients will react to more and more foods causing a greater imbalance of the immune system.

In my clinical practice the majority of the patients that I see have some form of gut dysfunction. Now there could be many reasons for this. I believe that it is due to the effects of the modern diet, particularly the consumption of high glycemic index carbohydrates or sugars. However, other explanations could include that I am now more aware of the role of gut function in chronic disease than I was in the past, or maybe I am attracting patients with gut problems based on my success in resolving these problems.

But the good news is that while there is an increase in the incidence of asthma, by understanding and correcting these causative factors it is possible to heal the gut, stabilize the immune system and therefore, reduce the frequency and severity of asthma for many patients.

Fish

Other nutrition changes that can increase the likelihood of getting asthma include the reduced amount of fish in diets. One of the studies that I came across recently showed that people who ate fish two or more times a week had a 30% less risk of getting asthma. That's a pretty powerful thing. A third of patients with asthma wouldn't get it if they just ate fish two or more times a week.

My Inhalers Are Very Good. But Is there Anything Else I Should Do?

The current medications for asthma are great. The modern inhalers include relievers, preventers and some of the newer long-acting agents. Most patients with asthma find an inhaler that works well for them. Anyone that has moderate to severe asthma, should have an action plan that describes what to do when their asthma gets worse. This would include increasing the dose of their inhalers through to calling an ambulance. This is a very important part of managing asthma.

Complement Your Inhalers

There are also some steps you can take yourself to gain better control of your asthma. Fish oils have been shown to reduce the risk of asthma. In fact, if you eat fish twice a week you lower your risk of asthma by 30%. However, even in established asthma, therapeutic levels of fish oils can reduce the irritability of the airways and for that reason they should be taken along-side asthma medications, unless you have a fish oil allergy.

While the essential fatty acids in fish oils are beneficial for asthma, the majority of fish oil supplements are stabilized with vitamin E which is obtained from a soy source. Some patients with asthma have a high level of allergies, and soy is a highly allergenic food. So if you have a soy allergy, you need to be careful about the fish oil that you take.

Probiotics contain good bacteria that assist us to have good health. They have been shown to balance the immune system, which we know from above is one of the causes of asthma. Studies have shown benefits of taking probiotics in patients with asthma.

This Lady's Asthma Improved After Probiotics

To demonstrate this, let me tell you the story of one of my clinic patients. Initially, her doctor sent her to me because she was getting a lot of bloating and other gut issues that did not respond to conventional treatment. She also has a very serious lung condition called pulmonary aspergillosus as well as asthma. With this patient, we started by making some preliminary dietary changes and used some key nutrients to improve gut function. She noticed an immediate improvement in stomach bloating and energy levels. When the results of her food sensitivity tests came back they showed severe reactions to eggs of which she was eating quite a lot. So we removed eggs from her diet and she achieved a more sustained improvement in energy levels. However, things still weren't quite right. So we investigated the balance of her gut bacteria using some specialized testing from a laboratory in the USA. I must confess that it was an omission of mine not to address her balance of good and bad bacteria at one of her earlier consultations.

Anyway, we started her on a preparation of lactobacillus only, since she had unusually high levels of bifidobacteria already. The improvements since have been quite dramatic. The last conversation I had with this patient was that she had so much energy that she was planning to do the Rangitoto swim. For those that don't know, this is an ocean swim from Rangitoto Island back to mainland Auckland which is about 5km. A big effort for anyone, but especially someone with asthma. Interestingly, she also commented that she has not needed her inhalers recently.

So while I didn't intentionally start out to improve this lady's asthma, balancing her immune system with probiotics certainly resulted in overall health improvement, including her asthma.

A Biochemisty Lesson

Researchers have found that there are a number of changes in important chemicals in people with asthma. One important chemical called cyclic AMP (cAMP) has been found to be present in much reduced amounts in patients with asthma. This is important because one of the known effects of cAMP is to relax smooth muscle, including the muscles lining the airways. So if you have low levels of cAMP, you will have smaller air passages due to the muscle surrounding the airway tubes being tight. Obviously, this is going to reduce airflow and make breathing more difficult.

So How Do We Increase cAMP Levels?

We know that there are a number of nutrients that can increase cAMP levels, including a number of herbs and the nutrient quercetin. Quercetin is actually present in a number of herbs, but is also found in berries, fruits and vegetables. So once again this is another reason to eat lots of fresh fruit (especially berries) and vegetables. I should also mention that green tea contains quercetin, so swapping green tea for your coffee should provide you with extra quercetin, which may improve your asthma.

Quercetin is interesting because in addition to increasing cAMP levels it will also decrease the production of lipoxygenase (LOX). Now I'm not trying to impress you with big biochemical names, there is a very important reason why I mention LOX. LOX is an enzyme in the body that produces a whole bunch of inflammatory products particularly in people with asthma. The products that come from LOX are the most potent chemical mediators in asthma. In fact, some of these chemicals are 1000 times more potent than histamine in stimulating the airways. Most people will know from bee stings, just how powerful histamine is in causing inflammation. So 1000 times stronger than histamine is a very strong effect indeed. In other words, people with asthma have high levels of LOX and high levels of inflammation. Taking quercetin can help to lower the levels of LOX, which should dramatically reduce inflammation in the airways.

Beware Of These Common Medicines

If you will allow me to complicate the biochemistry just one more bit, I'll describe an important reason why people with asthma should avoid one of the most common classes of medicines that is freely available. These medicines are even available from locations that do not have any medical supervision, e.g. supermarkets and petrol stations. That is dangerous if you ask me.

The NSAIDs are a group of medicines that are commonly used to relieve pain and fever. Common names for drugs in this class are ibuprofen (which you may know by the brand name Nurofen), diclofenac (Voltaren) or aspirin. I am sure you will have heard of them and will likely even have some in your medicine cabinet.

These powerful anti-inflammatory medicines work by reducing the production of another enzyme called cyclooxygenase (COX) and increasing the levels of LOX. In other words, by taking ibuprofen or diclofenac or any other similar pain killers, you'll get more LOX, and therefore you could get a real worsening of your asthma. What this means is that if you have asthma, you need to be very careful about taking those particular painkillers.

What Readily Available Substance Do Hospitals Use For Emergency Asthma Treatment?

No, hospitals don't use some fancy modern high-tech drug. They use plain old magnesium for people with severe asthma attacks. They will often give patients with a severe asthma attack an infusion of magnesium straight into their veins, which is just about 100% effective in resolving asthma. That is all very nice for the hospitals, but what does that mean for patients with mild to moderate asthma?

The important lesson here is that oral forms of magnesium can build up the body's stores of magnesium just as well as intravenous infusions. It just takes a little longer to build up levels in the bloodstream and then into cells, but an oral magnesium supplement will raise magnesium body levels.

Magnesium Supplementation

Magnesium works mostly inside your cells. In fact, 99% of your magnesium is located inside your cells and only about 1% is in the blood. Therefore, the amount of magnesium you've got in your bloodstream is not a good indicator of what's actually in the cells. However, increasing the level of magnesium in your blood allows it to quickly move into the cells. Furthermore, patients with chronic obstructive pulmonary disease have been shown to have low levels of magnesium in their muscles, despite having normal blood levels of magnesium.

So be careful if your doctor wants to do a magnesium blood test before recommending magnesium. They need to do a red blood cell magnesium level, not a serum level to truly assess what might be inside your cells.

It is a really good option for patients with asthma to take a magnesium supplement. Not only for the benefits in asthma, but for the many other health benefits that magnesium can provide. In fact, the list of what magnesium is good for could fill a book on its own! Magnesium is quite safe to take and many New Zealanders are deficient in magnesium.

We have already mentioned that blood tests for magnesium levels are not accurate. But there are many physical signs and symptoms that would indicate you have a magnesium deficiency. If your pharmacist is trained in nutrition medicine, then they will be able to provide you with a check list of symptoms that can help you know whether you have a magnesium deficiency or not.

Some of these symptoms include irritability, anxiety, agitation, restlessness, insomnia, noise intolerance, hyperactivity, confusion, dizziness, palpitations, heart arrhythmia, high blood pressure, poor circulation with cold hands and feet, muscle twitching and cramps, tremors, muscle soreness, headache, anorexia, fatigue, and depression. In fact there are over 300 different enzymes in the body that need magnesium to work properly!

Selenium Deficiency Has Also Been Linked to Asthma

Low selenium levels have been observed in New Zealanders with asthma. If you were paying attention a little earlier in the book, you will remember the importance of LOX in asthma. Selenium helps to control the LOX pathway, and protects cells against damage. So this might be a mechanism for the way selenium can help with asthma. We know that New Zealand soil is deficient in selenium, so it would be worthwhile for patients with asthma to supplement their diets with a bit of selenium as well as magnesium. In theory, too much selenium can be toxic, so it would be best to talk to your pharmacist about how much selenium you should take. It will depend on how much you might be getting from other sources such as your diet or from multivitamins.

Other signs of a deficiency of selenium include high cholesterol levels, poor pancreatic enzyme production, impaired liver function, recurrent infections, and male sterility. Recent evidence suggests that selenium deficiency increases the risk of cancer and arteriosclerosis. Signs of selenium toxicity include hair loss, brittle nails, yellowish skin, pallor, skin eruptions, lassitude, fatigue, arthritis, muscle pains, diabetes, liver damage, kidney damage, immune system depression, anorexia, abdominal discomfort and pain, garlic-breath odor, metallic taste in mouth, muscle paralysis, coma and death.

What Drugs Should Asthmatics Avoid?

We talked about the pain-killing medicines called the NSAIDs earlier, and how they can cause an increase in LOX and all the associated inflammatory reactions that can worsen asthma. Therefore the NSAIDs should be avoided in someone with severe or moderate asthma. I guess then the painkiller of choice for people with asthma would be paracetamol. Now I don't want to seem like a party-pooper, but patients with asthma should be cautioned about taking paracetamol too. Paracetamol will reduce the amount of another enzyme in the body called glutathione peroxidase, which is a very strong anti-oxidant enzyme that normally protects the body. We know there is a lot of oxidative damage going on in asthma, so patients with asthma really need all the protection they can get.

If you are in a lot of pain you need to take something, and so paracetamol would be the preferred option. If the pain is only mild then maybe think about being cautious about taking paracetamol. And if you need to take paracetamol on a fairly regular basis, then you should talk to your pharmacist about what you can do to boost your anti-oxidant levels because that will help to overcome the side effects of paracetamol.

Beta-Blockers And Asthma

There is a common medication for blood pressure called beta blockers and they work by blocking the beta receptors in the heart as the name suggests. However, they may also block the beta receptors in lungs, which can cause narrowing in the airways. In fact, the most common inhalers contain salbutamol (Ventolin), which actually stimulates beta receptors. In other words, they work in exactly the opposite way to these blood pressure medications. So if you have asthma and your doctor is considering putting you on blood pressure medications too, just make sure that you remind him or her about your asthma. Alternatively, ask your pharmacist if there are any interactions between all your medicines for asthma and blood pressure.

Theophylline Nutrient Interactions

There are a number of medications that can be used for asthma, which reduce the levels of key nutrients in the body. We call these drug-nutrient interactions. Theophylline (brand name Nuelin) is not used that commonly these days, but it certainly has an effect on your nutrient status. In particular, theophylline can reduce the levels of vitamin B6, which can result in a lot of toxicity. When you take theophylline, the main side effects include headaches, nausea, irritability, and being unable to sleep, which all disappear if you take vitamin B6. So patients with asthma who have been prescribed theophylline should take a good B-vitamin complex.

Steroids And Nutrient Problems

The corticosteroids are one of the most common treatments for asthma. They are used in "preventer" inhalers and are also used in tablet form (such as prednisone tablets) when asthma is bad. These medications can reduce the levels of a few nutrients in your body including vitamin A, vitamin C, vitamin B6, folate, potassium, calcium, and phosphorus. So it would be worthwhile asking your pharmacist about what you need to do to recoup those nutrients into your body. The answer to that question would depend on the symptoms that you may be experiencing and the strength of the steroid medication that you are taking. You may be able to get away with a high quality multivitamin supplement or you may need some specific higher dose nutrients to make sure that you avoid the side effects of the steroid medications.

If I Supplement My Asthma Medications Will I Feel A Difference?

The response that people get from supplements (and medicines too) will vary between individuals. Perhaps the best way to describe the results that are possible from supplementing your asthma medications is for me to tell you about James who was one of my patients. James had had asthma all his life. He is 29 years old, plays rugby, was told by his doctor to change his diet and lifestyle as he had borderline high blood pressure. If James couldn't get his blood pressure down by healthy living, the doctor was going to have to put him on blood pressure medications. James didn't really want to go down that track and it's great that his doctor gave him a chance to improve his blood pressure rather than jumping straight to prescription drugs. He came to me to help him get his blood pressure down naturally. Now, when patients come to see me in my clinic, I don't just treat the first problem they identify. Instead, I like to assemble all the information that might help me figure out what metabolic processes might not be working properly. In doing so, I am more likely to discover the cause of the problem rather than treat one symptom of it.

As part of my case history that I took from James, I discovered he had a lot of joint pains, which he just put down to getting old (at 29 years of age!). He also thought it was related to being a rugby player and giving his body a "hammering" every week. We also noticed that he started putting on a little bit of weight particularly around his middle. Fat around the stomach ("beer gut") is not uncommon for a male. This gut fat is more dangerous than fat elsewhere in the body because it is metabolically active fat. So I advised him on a change of diet, including modifying his alcohol intake which was one of the big factors wrong with his diet. We put him on fish oils, magnesium, CoQ10, and some high strength anti-oxidants, in an attempt to improve his blood pressure. After a few months his blood pressure did improve which was great. But what we also noticed was that he had lost weight and his asthma improved. In fact, his asthma improved to a level that he didn't need his Ventolin inhalers during his rugby games.

So James' story had a nice happy ending. I think the reason that we got an improvement in his asthma was by significantly reducing the inflammation in his body by a low-inflammatory diet and the anti-inflammatory effects of his supplements.

10

Arthritis

Are Anti-Inflammatories Bad For You?

A major factor in arthritis is the presence of inflammation, which means pain, swelling, heat and redness, especially in joints. So if you stop the inflammation, you pretty much stop the arthritis. For this reason, anti-inflammatory medicines are not bad. We have mentioned some nutrients earlier in this book that reduce inflammation and are quite safe to use. However, some anti-inflammatory medications do have potentially serious side effects.

The main anti-inflammatory medicines used in arthritis are called NSAIDs (non-steroidal anti-inflammatory drugs). These include medicines such as ibuprofen, diclofenac and naproxen, which are anti-inflammatories that you can buy over the counter without a prescription. In fact, ibuprofen can be purchased from a supermarket! Because these medicines are freely available, we tend to forget just how serious their side effects can be.

The Scary Truth About NSAIDs

In fact, an article in the American Journal of Medicine indicated that there were over 100,000 people hospitalized, and over 16,000 deaths every year from the gastrointestinal side effects of NSAIDs in arthritis patients. The authors commented that this was a conservative estimate. Just to be clear, these were patients who were taking these anti-inflammatory drugs in the recommended therapeutic doses, not patients who had overdosed. I personally think it is frightening that you can buy these medications from a supermarket or petrol station without any supervision from trained medical people.

A Pain In The Gut

The NSAIDs irritate the gut lining, which can result in bleeding and serious side effects. But there are also mild effects that may go unnoticed but which may cause a low level of continual damage that in the end can be quite devastating. For example, gut function can be impaired, which as we know from previous chapters can give rise to inflammation in the body.

So you can see that NSAIDs can potentially cause the problem that they are being used to treat. In other words, NSAIDs can actually make arthritis worse in the long term, even though they are relieving some of the symptoms in the short term.

NSAIDs And Your Kidneys

In addition to stomach problems, NSAIDs have also been associated with kidney failure. Kidney function tends to decline with age, so it's not surprising that elderly patients can have major kidney problems after taking NSAIDS.

In fact, one gerontologist from the USA that I used to work with would not put patients over the age of 65 on NSAIDs. I questioned him about whether this was an over-reaction and suggested that we just monitor their kidney function and stop the NSAIDs if any changes started to happen.

However, he was adamant that patients over 65 years of age should never take NSAIDs because the effect on kidney function can be very rapid (i.e. within a week or two) and very serious. So we should exercise a lot of caution before using these medicines.

One Medicine Can Lead To Many More

Because of the potential for NSAIDs to damage the gut, they are commonly given with another class of drugs that are intended to help protect the stomach. The most common gut protecting medicines are the proton pump inhibitors (PPIs) which you may know by names like omeprazole (Losec) or pantoprazole (Somac), or lansoprazole (Solox). These medicines do help to thicken up the lining of the stomach, and do relieve the symptoms of heart burn and reflux for many patients. But they are associated with long term health problems.

And Many Medicines Can Lead To Poor Health

One of the most important problems with the PPIs is that they increase the risk of getting irritable bowel syndrome (diarrhoea and/or constipation). They work by reducing stomach acid very strongly, which relieves the symptoms of heart burn but increases the chance of inflammatory changes in the body. However, stomach acid is important for digestion. So by reducing acid production, you can get impaired digestion and subsequent inflammation in the gastrointestinal tract leading to irritable bowel syndrome. It can also mean that you are more likely to get nutrient deficiencies.

For example, minerals need acid to be digested, it is called acidification. Take magnesium as an important mineral to consider. If you have low levels of stomach acid, you will subsequently have low levels of magnesium, which could lead to muscle tightness and muscle cramping. For patients who have arthritis, these muscle problems can put stress on the skeleton and aggravate the existing bone and joint pain.

Alternatives To NSAIDs

There are alternative products that can provide pain relief and anti-inflammatory effects. The good news is that these alternative anti-inflammatories are gut friendly, which means you get the same relief without the increased risk of poor health in the future. We recommend a number of herbs in our clinic and pharmacy to reduce inflammation. There are some good combination products that contain therapeutic doses of the anti-inflammatory herbs. You can also add them to your cooking for extra effect. Useful herbs that are commonly available as food flavourings that would be good to consider include turmeric, ginger and cayenne pepper.

The Latest Medicines Can Have Problems Too

The problem with the side effects of anti-inflammatory drugs is so serious that the pharmaceutical industry has spent billions of dollars developing new medicines that would not have such side effects. However, most have been withdrawn because they have been found to increase the risk of heart attack and stroke. The remaining ones have been reserved for patients who really need them and who cannot tolerate other anti-inflammatory medicines. So they are not prescribed very frequently. Interestingly, my father with all his arthritis complaints has been on most oral anti-inflammatory drugs for 40-plus years. He has had a number of stomach bleeds and ulcers through that time and had a stroke a few years ago. It would be impossible to say what caused his stroke, but the combination of all the medicines and the high level of inflammation in his body would increase his risk of stroke.

Some Great New High Cost Medicines

Not all of the new medicines are bad. Several new arthritis drugs have been developed that act on specific immune cells like TNF-alpha and IgG1. Humira is one of these medicines. These are highly targeted drugs and most need to be taken by injection. The reports that I have received from patients who are taking these injections have been very positive. However, because of their cost (several thousand dollars each month), their availability has been restricted, so only people meeting certain criteria are given prescriptions for them.

And Low Cost Alternatives

If you don't meet the criteria to get these new drugs, it is comforting to know that there are low cost alternatives. Nutrients that have been shown to reduce levels of TNF-alpha include fish oils, zinc, cats claw, ginger, barley grass, quercetin, and green tea. Now these agents might not be as specific and as powerful as drugs like Humira, but when used as part of a balanced approach to arthritis and inflammation, they can provide substantial improvement in symptoms.

In other words, these nutrients have similar actions as the latest pharmaceutical injection that costs thousands of dollars per injection.

What Can We Do To Decrease The Side Effects Of Arthritis Drugs?

Some people need to take some form of anti-inflammatory medication. Their pain and their inflammation are so strong that they just need to do it. Otherwise, they might not be able to get out of bed. There is a lot that can be done to investigate the causes of their inflammation and then treat those underlying causes. But in the meantime, they need relief for their pain and inflammation. So for these people we need to protect the gut. There are medications that are traditionally prescribed to do that, such as the proton pump inhibitors (PPIs) like omeprazole. However, the PPIs are associated with a lot of side effects as I've mentioned in the previous chapters on digestion. My preference would be to use a number of safer and better tolerated gut protectants like glutamine, aloe vera, slippery elm, quercetin and even licorice, which all help to protect the stomach against the effects of the NSAIDs.

How Do We Treat The Side Effects Of The Medicines For The Side Effects Of The Medicines?

The heading of this section is not a typo, but is a reasonably common observation when you work in a pharmacy. We often see patients taking medicines designed to treat the side effects of other medicines. Then they develop side effects to the second medication. Now I am not suggesting that this is the work of bad doctors. I believe it is a consequence of a time-poor health system that is focused on population-level, evidence-based medicine. As mentioned previously, while in theory this approach to medicine seems well intentioned, it can lead to an over-reliance on treatments that are developed by companies with large resources. You need to have strong financial power to run large-scale clinical trials required to collect the "evidence." In other words, it is an industry that has been dominated by the pharmaceutical companies.

But back to our problem of what you need to do if you take PPIs to protect your gut from the effects of the NSAIDs. The main problem with the use of PPIs is disruption of digestion, and the many health problems that stem from the impaired digestion. Therefore, to protect yourself from the adverse effects of the PPIs I would recommend a variety of nutrients that have the ability to enhance digestion. Patients taking PPIs generally have a reduction in the level of digestive enzymes produced from the pancreas. So supplementing with digestive enzymes is important. We would also want to protect the kidneys. There are a good few nutrients that will help this, CoQ10 would be one. In addition to helping with kidney function, CoQ10 will help strengthen the heart so while there is some evidence of a link between NSAIDs use and more heart disease, taking CoQ10 gives that underlying protection. These nutrients can prevent further medication-induced health problems.

My preference is to trial safer anti-inflammatory nutrients instead of the PPI medications. Most studies show that these nutrients are at least as effective as the conventional medications. In other words, rather than keep adding plasters over the open sore, it would be better to treat the cause of the sore, so that we need fewer plasters.

What Are Gut-Friendly Anti-Inflammatories?

There has been a lot of research on the anti-inflammatory effects of turmeric and one if its components called curcumin. You will probably be familiar with these substances, especially if you have ever cooked a curry. Some studies have shown that curcumin has equal anti-inflammatory effects to the NSAIDs, so that's really positive. However, curcumin is not well absorbed orally, so you need to take quite high doses to have an effect. In other words, a good curry is probably not going to give you a full therapeutic dose, instead you might need to take supplements. Curcumin has been shown to have protective effects on the gut, as does zinc.

Zinc in high doses has strong anti-inflammatory effects. In fact, if you really push the dose up to very high levels you can get suppression of the immune system. However, your nutrition medicine pharmacist can provide you with great advice to avoid any possible problems from taking too much zinc.

MSM is a natural sulfa-based anti-inflammatory medication. Several books have been written about the benefits of MSM. Not only is it available in capsule form to help with joint and muscle aches and pains, but it is also available in creams to rub on sore areas and even nasal sprays to help reduce sinus pain and swelling.

The omega 3 fatty acids will help to balance the immune system and reduce inflammation. However, the anti-inflammatory effects of these fish oils do not happen quickly like they do with curcumin. The effects can take a little bit of time. This delay in effect reflects the time it takes for the omega 3 fatty acids to get incorporated into the new cell membranes. In other words, the fish oils are not something you use in a situation like "I've got a sore leg today, I'll take some fish oils to fix it." It's more of a long term strategy of preventing that inflammation in your body.

Interestingly we have mentioned the role of supplements of pancreatic digestive enzymes in improving digestion. However, they are also really helpful as anti-inflammatory agents in their own right, but only if they are taken between meals. The presence of food does influence their action. If you take the enzymes just before you eat, they will assist with digestion. If you take them on an empty stomach (at least an hour or two away from food) they will reduce inflammation. In fact, taking pancreatic enzymes between meals is a very powerful way of reducing inflammation in the body. With these herbs and nutrients, the dosage and the timing is quite important so you need to talk to your nutrition medicine-trained pharmacist about the best way of safely treating your pain and inflammation.

What Else Should I Do To Improve My Arthritis?

If you really want to put the time and the effort in to improving your arthritis then you should change to a low-inflammatory diet. Changing diet requires commitment and dedication, as eating is more than just nutrition, there is a great social aspect to it. This is especially so when we consider alcohol. So if you are not prepared to take time and effort, then changing your diet is not for you. However, if you are willing to make changes, then you will be assured of great results.

In our Nutrition Medicine Clinic we usually achieve great benefits from improving a patient's diet. We always start with a diet first because a lot of the inflammation in the body comes from eating inflammatory foods, which are very common today.

For example, most people have a very high level of omega-6 fatty acids. These fatty acids result in the production of inflammatory chemicals. Historically, we evolved on a diet that had a one-to-one balance of the omega-6 to the omega-3 fatty acids. In other words, we had a balance of inflammatory and anti-inflammatory chemicals in the body. Now, the ratio has shifted to 20-to-1. Put another way, we have 20 times the amount of inflammatory molecules running around in our bodies than anti-inflammatory ones. Obviously this can contribute to the development of inflammatory diseases, such as arthritis.

When Good Foods Cause Bad Problems

An increasing number of people are realizing that food "allergies" are a cause of ill health. I put the word "allergies" in inverted commas because not all food reactions meet the medical definition of an allergy. Sometimes foods cause sensitivities, which means when eaten they produce adverse effects, even if they do not produce the conventional changes needed to be classified as an allergy. Often these food sensitivities are associated with normally healthy foods, such as dairy, wheat, fish, nuts, soy and eggs. The saying *"One man's meat is another man's poison"* is quite accurate in this instance.

Just Plain Bad Foods

While some good foods can cause bad problems in sensitive people, there are other foods that I have found from experience with my patients in my clinic that are not good for anyone. Gluten is one that is worth a mention. Gluten is a protein composite that is contained in wheat and some other grains. It is also used as an additive in other foods to increase the protein levels and to assist with "glueing" it together. Studies in healthy young men have shown that after eating gluten, inflammatory changes in the gut are observed. Just to make it clear, these were healthy young men. Imagine what it can do to people who already have inflammation!

Call me a party pooper if you want, but alcohol causes problems in the gut. Studies have shown that intestinal permeability, which is a risk factor for inflammation and poor health, is increased for two weeks after consuming alcohol. So if you drink alcohol once every two weeks, you will likely have some level of increased intestinal permeability.

Am I A Bad Father?

A good illustration of the effects of gluten and alcohol is the case of my son. By the age of 18, he was getting regular "tummy bugs." In other words diarrhea and vomiting. He was also becoming "a little difficult" to live with. I tried to talk to him about the possible effects of his diet on his health, but this just fell on deaf ears. I should add that he was a big cheese roll fan. Once the pain and inconvenience of his condition got too much for him, my wife took him to see our local Chiropractor. The Chiropractor tested him for reactions to food and suggested that he stop gluten, dairy and beer.

At first, it was like the world was ending. Imagine trying to feed a very sporty and hungry 18 year old male without his staple food sources (cheese rolls). After two weeks, I thought that to avoid a murder charge either he was going to have to move out of home or the rest of the family might have to move into protective custody (maybe I'm exaggerating just a bit!). But then the changes started to kick in. He started to feel the increase in energy. He had gone several weeks without a "tummy bug." We noticed that he started being communicative and chatty. Instead of drawing straws with my wife to see who was going to talk to him (and risk a verbal beating in the process), we began to look forward to having very pleasant conversations with him. He even started initiating the conversations himself. Now he is a dedicated follower of a gluten-free diet, because he knows just what a difference it makes to his health. So much so that even when he is with his mates and they all go to Burger King or Wendys, he will not stray off his diet. When it comes to alcohol, he has managed to find some drinks that he can tolerate in moderation. There have been a few big "binges" that have slipped in over the last year, and predictably he has paid the price for that. But he is a teenager, so you can't spoil all his fun.

I often think that a good father would have been more assertive about the effects of diet on his health. Instead, it was our local Chiropractor that got the message home. I guess that is an example of how difficult it is to treat your own family. Sometimes it is better to hear these messages from an independent person, not your dad.

Digestion: The Next Frontier

If improving diet is the first step to stopping arthritis, then the second step is to improve digestion. You may ask what does digestion have to do with arthritis? If you're not digesting your food properly, your big proteins don't get broken down into the amino acids that your body needs to work properly. Plus these undigested proteins are not recognized by your body's defense force and so they get treated as foreign invaders by your immune system. Therefore, because of poor digestion your body produces a whole lot of inflammatory "protective" chemicals that run around your body and end up attacking your own tissues, such as attacking your knee joint or your hip joint or your fingers. So improving your digestion will reduce those big peptides and proteins from causing damage throughout the body.

More Arthritis Means Less Hormones

There are a number of reasons why patients with arthritis tend to get frail as they get older. There is the obvious reason that they often don't do as much exercise as other people and therefore their muscles start to shrink. Patients with arthritis also frequently have poor digestion as mentioned above, so they don't absorb the protein that they need to maintain their muscles. In other words, they don't use or feed their muscles properly.

An often overlooked factor in patients with arthritis is that they also tend to have an imbalance of their hormone levels. People with arthritis have a lot of inflammation, which is a stressful state for the body. To cope with this stress, the body produces a greater amount of stress hormones such as cortisol. However, this usually means that there is a correspondingly reduced production of the anabolic (muscle building) hormones such as testosterone and DHEA.

Hormone Imbalance Contributes To Poor Health

Testosterone is an important "feel good" hormone for both men and women. Testosterone is broken down by an enzyme in your body called aromatase. When you have a lot of inflammation in your body, the amount of aromatase increases. Therefore, you are more likely to have a shortage of testosterone. A shortage of testosterone has been documented to cause a whole lot more aches and pains, as well as feelings of irritability, bad mood, inability to concentrate, and problems with libido or sex drive. That doesn't sound like the kind of person I want to be. Who wants to be a grumpy, moody, person with lots of aches and pains and poor concentration? Heck, forget about the low sex drive, no-one like that is going to find a partner to begin with!

Like a lot of processes in the body, it becomes a bit of a vicious spiral. Inflammation disrupts hormone balance, and the hormone imbalance causes more aches and pains. By knowing the effects of hormones on the well-being of patients with arthritis, you can test the levels and use supplements where indicated. It is complicated, so it's important to consult a nutrition medicine-trained pharmacist so that you can get that whole picture and treat the actual causes of your inflammation and not just mask the symptoms with painkillers.

Martin: The Cured Arthritis Sufferer

A good case that illustrates the successful treatment of arthritis is me. I've already mentioned my story, but let me go over the highlights (or low lights) to illustrate my point. I developed ankylosing spondylitis (a form of arthritis) about 15 years ago. At that time I had a diet that was very high in inflammatory foods. You may ask why a pharmacist would eat a poor diet. Well, I actually didn't know it was a poor diet. I thought I was eating a healthy diet. All the messages from the conventional dietary experts told me to 'cut the fat'. So cut the fat I did. What I ended up doing was having a diet that was very high in inflammatory carbohydrates, had very little of the good essential fatty acids, and was very low in protein as well. So that had an impact on my whole digestive function and it may be why I subsequently developed a milk allergy.

But through my research associated with my studies in nutrition medicine I learned what I really should have been eating to ensure good health. I first worked on tidying up my diet, mainly by ensuring a high level of the good fats and quality proteins. I get a lot of good quality fats from fish, for example. I've reduced my intake of grains and inflammatory carbohydrates. I've taken milk out of my diet because my body reacts to that.

I used supplements to replace my stomach acid to improve my digestion. I used supplements of pancreatic enzymes, so I could digest my food better. The nutrients that I have used in fairly high doses include fish oils, magnesium and zinc. Once I started to feel my aches, pains and joint stiffness were gone, I started to think about getting really well. I now give myself a boost with coenzyme Q10 that helps to protect my heart, but also just gives me great energy because I live my life to the full with my work as a pharmacist and a nutrition medicine practitioner, writing books, speaking engagements, my family life, plus I do a lot of sports as well. If you need an energy boost and have never tried coenzyme Q10, I would recommend giving it a go. However, some brands are far superior to others when it comes to coenzyme Q10, and it can interact with some other medications. So, please make sure you consult your pharmacist before buying a bottle.

I provide you with my story so you can see that you can change disease outcomes by altering your diet and through careful use of supplements. You don't have to accept that just because your father had arthritis and so did your father's father, that you must necessarily suffer from the same condition. There are safe and natural solutions available for you to fight back.

11

Other Conditions

This Could Be A Book That Never Ends

My goal in writing this book was to make people aware that to achieve full health and vitality requires more than just conventional medicine.

This book was never intended to be a definitive text on all conditions and the ideal treatment strategies for them. Such a book would never get finished since there is always new information and research being published. Instead, I used a few of the most common conditions to illustrate how a sensible combined approach using conventional and complementary medicines can help achieve great health results.

If your condition is not one of the ones I have listed then I suggest that you talk to your optimal prescription health-trained pharmacist to help you filter out the good information from the bad. Alternatively, you could book in for a free Nutricheck Health Analysis (see the offer in the front of the book).

A Nutricheck Health Analysis can help you discover:

- how likely it is that your health condition is actually caused by a low level of one or more nutrients

- what nutrients your body is crying out for

- if your prescription medicines have caused low levels of essential nutrients.

Complementing Your Prescription: What About My Condition

As mentioned in the previous section this book is not intended to be the definitive text book on how to obtain optimal health outcomes from every prescription medicine. I do hope to alert people to the fact that there is more to health than just their prescription medicine. In other words, I am trying to *"teach you to fish"* rather than *"give you a fish."*

But to help you on your way I'll summarise some of the nutrient problems that can arise from common medicines (see table). You need to remember that any nutrient deficiencies can cause the body to work less efficiently. If left for too long, then some processes in the body can even stop working. I have a software package that tests for nutrient deficiencies, and my sickest patients always show up with the most deficiencies. My experience with patients in my clinic is that once you correct these deficiencies, the improvement in their health begins very quickly. I guess what I am saying is that these nutrient deficiencies should be taken very seriously if you want to ensure good health.

For your convenience I have drawn up a table of common medicines and the nutrients that they might affect. I have also included the common side effects of these medicines.

Nutrient Imbalances Caused By Common Medicines

Caution! You should not self medicate with the nutrients affected as listed. For some medicines there is an increased level of these nutrients and for some there is a decreased level of these nutrients. For medicines with a narrow range between effective dose and toxic dose, then supplementing with nutrients may cause toxicity. You should speak to your trusted health professional before taking any supplements with your medicines. Medications are listed by their generic name. Your prescription may be labelled with a brand name. Ask your pharmacist for the generic name of your medicine if you want to use this list.

Drug	Nutrients Affected	Associated Adverse Effect
ACE Inhibitors (captopril, quinapril, enalapril)	Potassium, Zinc	Nausea, vomiting, constipation, diarrhoea, reduced appetite, altered taste, dry mouth.
Alendronate (Fosamax)	Calcium, vitamin D	Nausea, vomiting, constipation, diarrhoea, alerted taste, difficulty swallowing.
Amphotericin (Fungilin)	Potassium, magnesium, zinc.	Nausea, vomiting, diarrhoea, reduced weight and appetite.
Antacids	Potassium, calcium, iron, phosphate, copper, B12, folate, C.	Nausea, vomiting, increased weight (fluid accumulation), reduced appetite, increased thirst.
Antibiotics	Good bacteria, vitamin K, Vitamin C, calcium, magnesium	Nausea, vomiting, diarrhoea, muscle cramps and twitches, irritability, anxiety, mood changes, immune system impairment, allergies.
Bendrofluazide	Potassium, magnesium, zinc, calcium, sodium	Nausea, vomiting, constipation, diarrhoea, reduced appetite, dry mouth, thirst.
Calcium	Iron	Reduced appetite, altered taste, dry mouth.
Carbamazepine	Vitamin B6, folate, biotin, Vitamin D, Vitamin K, carnitine	Nausea, vomiting, constipation, diarrhoea, weight changes, appetite changes, altered taste, dry mouth.
Carbimazole	Iron, Iodine, selenium, lithium, vitamin A	Nausea, vomiting, diarrhoea, weight loss, appetite changes, itchy skin.
Cholestyramine	Magnesium, zinc, calcium, iron, vitamin B12, folate, vitamins K, E, D and A.	Nausea, vomiting, constipation, diarrhoea, weight changes, reduced appetite, altered taste, difficulty swallowing.
Colchicine	Potassium, calcium, sodium, iron, vitamin B12, vitamin A.	Nausea, vomiting, diarrhoea, reduced weight and appetite.
Dexamethasone	Potassium, zinc, calcium, phosphate, chromium, vitamin B6, folate, vitamin C, vitamin D, vitamin A	Nausea, vomiting, increased weight, appetite changes.

Drug	Nutrients Affected	Associated Adverse Effect
Digoxin	Potassium, magnesium, Calcium	Nausea, vomiting, diarrhoea, reduced weight, reduced appetite.
Furosemide	Potassium, magnesium, zinc, calcium, sodium, chloride	Nausea, vomiting, diarrhoea, reduced appetite, dry mouth, thirst.
Glibenclamide	Iodine	Nausea, vomiting, constipation, diarrhoea, increased weight and appetite changes.
Gliclazide	Iodine	Nausea, vomiting, constipation, diarrhoea, increased weight and appetite changes.
Haloperidol	Vitamin B2, vitamin B12	Nausea, vomiting, constipation, diarrhoea, weight changes, appetite changes, altered taste, dry mouth, salivation.
Hydrocortisone	Potassium, zinc, calcium, phosphate, chromium, vitamin B6, folate, vitamin C, vitamin D, vitamin A	Nausea, vomiting, increased weight, appetite changes.
Indapamide	Potassium, magnesium, sodium	Nausea, vomiting, constipation, diarrhoea, reduced weight, reduced appetite, dry mouth.
Laxatives	Potassium, magnesium, calcium, sodium, vitamin K, Vitamin D	Nausea, rebound constipation, diarrhoea, reduced weight.
Levodopa	Vitamin B6, folate, vitamin C	Nausea, vomiting, constipation, diarrhoea, weight changes, reduced appetite, altered taste, no taste, dry mouth, increased saliva, difficulty swallowing.
Lithium carbonate	Sodium, copper, iodine	Nausea, vomiting, diarrhoa, weight changes, decreased appetite, altered taste, dry mouth, increased thirst, increased salivation.
Madopar	Vitamin B6, folate, vitamin C	Nausea, vomiting, constipation, diarrhoea, weight changes, reduced appetite, altered taste, dry mouth, difficulty swallowing.

Drug	Nutrients Affected	Associated Adverse Effect
Metformin	Vitamin B12, folate, glucose	Nausea, vomiting, constipation, diarrhoea, reduced weight, reduced appetite, altered taste.
Methotrexate	Calcium, vitamin B12, folate	Nausea, vomiting, diarrhoea, reduced weight, reduced appetite, altered taste.
NSAIDS (aspirin, ibuprofen, diclofenac)	Potassium, iron, B12, folate, vitamin C	Nausea, vomiting, reduced appetite.
Omeprazole	Iron, B1, B12, Magnesium, Calcium	Nausea, vomiting, constipation, diarrhoea, increased weight, altered taste, dry mouth, muscle cramps and twitches, irritability, anxiety, mood changes.
Oral Contraceptives	Magnesium, zinc, copper, vitamin B12, vitamin C, vitamin A, good bacteria	Nausea, vomiting, diarrhoea, weight changes, appetite changes.
Phenytoin	Magnesium, calcium, vitamin B6, folate, biotin, vitamin K, vitamin D	Nausea, vomiting, constipation, increased weight, reduced appetite, altered taste.
Potassium	Vitamin B12	Nausea, vomiting, diarrhoea.
Prednisone	Potassium, zinc, calcium, sodium, phosphate, chromium, vitamin B6, folate, vitamins C, D and A	Nausea, vomiting, constipation, diarrhoea, increased weight, appetite changes.
Primidone	Calcium, vitamin B6, folate, biotin, vitamin D, vitamin K	Nausea, vomiting, weight and appetite changes.
Promethazine	Vitamin B2	Nausea, vomiting, constipation, diarrhoea, reduced appetite, altered taste, dry mouth.
Proton Pump Inhibitors (omeprazole, pantroprazole, lansoprazole)	Iron, vitamin B1, vitamin B12, most minerals	Nausea, vomiting, constipation, diarrhoea, altered taste, dry mouth, various symptoms of mineral deficiency.

Drug	Nutrients Affected	Associated Adverse Effect
Ranitidine	Iron, B12, B1	Nausea, vomiting, constipation, diarrhoea, reduced appetite, dry mouth.
Ranitidine	Iron, vitamin B1, vitamin B12, most minerals	Nausea, vomiting, diarrhoea, constipation.
Sinemet	Vitamin B6, folate, vitamin C	Nausea, vomiting, constipation, diarrhoea, weight changes, reduced appetite, altered taste, dry mouth, difficulty swallowing.
Sodium valproate (Epilim)	Folate, biotin, vitamin D, carnitine	Nausea, vomiting, diarrhoea, increased weight, appetite changes.
Spironolactone	Potassium, calcium, magnesium, sodium	Nausea, vomiting, diarrhoea, reduced appetite, dry mouth, thirst.
SSRIs (Fluoxetine, paroxetine, citalopram)	Sodium	Nausea, vomiting, constipation, diarrhoea, increased weight, increased appetite, altered taste, dry mouth, thirst, increased salivation, difficulty swallowing.
Sulfasalazine	Iron, folate	Nausea, vomiting, diarrhoea, decreased appetite.
Thyroxine (levothyroxine)	Iron, Iodine, selenium, lithium, vitamin A	Nausea, vomiting, diarrhoea, reduced weight, appetite changes.
Tricyclic antidepressants (amitriptyline, nortriptyline)	B2	Nausea, vomiting, constipation, diarrhoea, weight changes, appetite changes, altered taste, dry mouth.
Warfarin	Vitamin K, vitamin E, vitamin D	Nausea, vomiting, diarrhoea.

As an extra bonus gift to you I have created for you a list of the common signs of nutrient deficiencies of some nutrients.

Possible Signs Of Nutrient Deficiency

Nutrient	Deficiency Signs
Vitamin B1	Apathy, confusion, emotional lability, depression, fatigue, insomnia, irritability, nervousness, headache, memory-loss, muscle weakness, increased pain-sensitivity, numbness/burning in the hands or feet, increased sound-sensitivity, indigestion, loss of appetite, constipation, sluggish metabolism, palpitations, shortness of breath and heart-failure.
Vitamin B2	Insomnia, dizziness and depression, light-sensitivity, red-itchy-burning eyes, blurred vision, cataracts, magenta-hued tongue, cheilosis (Cracks/soreness in corners of mouth), oily/scaly skin (especially around mouth and nose), dyssebacea (whiteheads and blackheads), acne, excessive hair loss.
Vitamin B3	Fearful feelings, anxiety, excessive worry, suspiciousness, feelings of gloom, depression, fatigue, irritability, insomnia, muscle tension/soreness, headaches, anorexia/nausea, abdominal discomfort/pain, flatulence/wind, bloating, halitosis, diarrhoea, muscle weakness, burning sensation in tongue & limbs, sensory dysperception, dementia, cognitive disorders, strawberry-tip tongue, white-coated tongue, mid-line cracks in tongue, dental-indentations at tongue margins, sore mouth, swollen/painful gums, dermatitis (localised scaly pigmented rash).
Vitamin B6	Nervousness, agitation, anxiety, emotional-upset, mood swings. Irritability, insomnia, depression, fatigue, poor dream-recall fluid-retention, premenstrual-tension, low blood sugar, low blood pressure, dizziness, acne (espec. post-adolescence), facial oiliness dandruff, hair-loss, cheilosis (cracks in mouth corners), sore tongue, anorexia and nausea, anaemia, numbness/tingling in hands/feet, impaired wound healing, arthritis (espec. in finger/toe joints).
Vitamin B5	Fatigue, exhaustion, depression, adrenal-exhaustion, anorexia, nausea/vomiting, abdominal bloating/discomfort, constipation burning feet, numbness/tingling in hands/feet, aching mid-back, impaired coordination, low blood pressure, Low blood sugar, recurrent infection, excessive hair-loss.

Nutrient	Deficiency Signs
Vitamin B12	Impaired memory, poor concentration, impaired learning, fatigue, depression, mood swings, mental illness leading to hallucinations, confusion, paranoia, psychosis, dizziness, numbness/tingling in hands/feet, unsteady gait and/or balance, red-sore-smooth tongue, poor digestion, abdominal discomfort.
Folate	Mental sluggishness, poor memory and concentration, apathy, fatigue, depression, paranoid-thinking, cheilosis, sore-red tongue, anorexia, poor digestion, constipation, shortness of breath, irritability, insomnia, restless legs. Folic acid deficiency in pregnancy is associated with foetal neural tube defects (Spina Bifida).
Biotin	Drowsiness, lassitude, apathy, depression, anorexia, nausea, muscle pains, excessive sensitivity to touch, skin rash (flaking, itchiness, grey-toned skin), anaemia, high cholesterol, hair-loss, pale-smooth tongue.
Vitamin C	Acute Deficiency: Sallow or muddy complexion, loss of vigor, lassitude, easily tired, impaired exercise tolerance, breathlessness, loss of appetite, anaemia, easy bruising, fleeting pains in joints and limbs (especially in legs).
Vitamin A	Impaired night-vision, aching and tired and burning eyes, inflamed eyelids, painful eyes, xeropthalmia, headaches, sinus congestion, recurrent URTI and flu-like illness, dry and flaky skin, lumpy skin (toad skin), acne-type skin lesions, dull and lustreless hair, ridged nails, peeling nails, impaired libido, breast soreness. Mental changes: Insomnia, fatigue, depression, neuralgia in limbs.
Vitamin D	Burning mouth and throat, scalp sweating (esp. at night), insomnia myopia, aching and sore eyes, muscle pain, muscle cramps, bone pain, deformed bone growth, easy fractures, nervousness anxiety, restlessness, hypothyroidism (underactive thyroid).
Vitamin E	Impaired circulation, cold and pale peripheries, disturbed nail growth, hyperkeratosis of heels, muscle soreness with exercise, tender calf muscles, muscle weakness, muscle wasting, fatigue, restless sleep, insomnia, dizziness, impaired balance, gait disturbance (ataxia), premenstrual syndrome (PMT), breast soreness, menopause symptoms, loss of libido, impotence. Increased tissue damage: premature ageing, cataracts, retinal degeneration, haemolytic anaemia, thrombocytosis. Increased risk of arteriosclerosis, heart disease and stroke, liver damage (cirrhosis), and senile dementia.

Nutrient	Deficiency Signs
Vitamin K	Increased bleeding tendency and easy bruising. Recent research suggests impaired blood sugar control may occur with inadequate Vitamin K.
Calcium	Irritability, anxiety, agitation, insomnia, poor memory, dizziness, palpitations, numbness, muscle-twitching, muscle cramps, convulsions, mental confusion, osteoporosis, rickets, tooth-decay and loss.
Magnesium	Irritability, anxiety, agitation, restlessness, insomnia, noise intolerance, hyperactivity, confusion, dizziness, palpitations, heart arrythmia, high blood pressure, poor circulation with cold hands and feet, muscle twitching and cramps, tremors, muscle soreness, headache, anorexia, fatigue, depression.
Sodium	Lassitude, muscle weakness, hot-weather fatigue, dizziness, low blood pressure, weak thready pulse, anorexia, abdominal cramps, nausea and vomiting, flatulence, headache, impaired memory, confusion, convulsions.
Potassium	Fatigue, anorexia, constipation, muscle weakness, muscle cramps, slow, palpitations, heart arrythmias, agitation, nervousness, depression.
Copper	Anaemia, alopecia, generalised weakness, fatigue, depression, skin rash, recurrent infection, diarrhoea, high cholesterol emphysema, osteopenia, myocardial degeneration.
Zinc	Acne, anorexia, loss of taste, eczema, glucose intolerance, diabetes, apathy, fatigue, depression, hyperactivity in children, impaired protein synthesis: hair loss, poor wound healing, skin stretch marks, soft or brittle nails, growing pains, recurrent infections, white-spots in nails, growth impairment: shortened stature, delayed sexual maturity, impotence, irregular menstruation.
Iron	Tiredness, easy fatigue, weakness, impaired memory, poor concentration, impaired cognitive ability, poor learning, depression, anaemia, dizziness, shortness of breath, cardiac failure, brittle nails, lustreless nails, flattened or spoon-shaped nails, hair loss, difficulty in swallowing.
Chromium	Mature-onset diabetes, high cholesterol levels, impaired growth, anxiety and fatigue.
Selenium	High cholesterol levels, poor pancreatic enzyme production, impaired liver function, recurrent infections, male sterility. Recent evidence suggests that selenium deficiency increases the risk of cancer and arteriosclerosis.

12

Ensuring You Get
The Best Care

Defusing The Fierce Debate:
Conventional Or Complementary?

I attend a lot of continuing education courses. Some are run by conventional medical organizations, and some by complementary medicine groups. Often there is reference made to the other profession, and sometimes the comments are disparaging. For example, the naturopaths might make reference to the misinformed doctors using dangerous drugs. Or the doctors might refer to the witch-doctor naturopath down the road using dangerous herbs.

The only people who get hurt by perpetuating these feelings are the patients. Each profession has some great tools at their disposal and if the professions would work together then the patient could experience the best of both worlds.

I sit on the fence since I have a knowledge and understanding of both conventional and complementary medicines. This way I can advise my patients about the best treatment plan for them.

There are medical practices starting to appear that are offering a combination of conventional and complementary medicine. However, there are still not enough of them to go around. In the meantime, I suggest understanding what questions to ask your healthcare provider to ensure you get the best possible treatment outcomes.

Why Your Pharmacist May Not Tell You What You Need To Get Well

There is an old management saying that states:

"No one gets up in the morning and says to themselves 'I'm going to do a really bad job at work today."

The lesson here is that people do generally try to do their best. However, sometimes people don't have the tools to do parts of their job properly. This is exactly the situation with many health professionals including doctors and pharmacists.

I was on a school camp last year with my youngest son, and I got talking to one of the other parent helpers who was a doctor. We started discussing the problematic patients that she sees in her practice. For some of these patients, there is no established effective medical therapy. In other words, she had no tools in her toolbox that were appropriate for such patients. I discussed the growing evidence from the field of nutrition medicine and how I did have some great tools to help these patients. We agreed it would make sense for us to work together to help these patients to get well.

The same goes for some pharmacists. Most pharmacists that I know are lovely caring people. But as a profession, we are taught very little about nutrition medicine at Pharmacy School. Since more than 70% of the causes of death are related to poor nutrition, this seems a major oversight by the Universities. So your pharmacist will not be able to help you if they haven't undertaken extra study outside of university.

Do You Want Fries With That?

The other big conflict that the pharmacy profession has to deal with is the issue of credibility and believability. In my pharmacy we always strive to educate people about their health and what they need to do to get the best outcomes from their medicines. Sometimes this involves recommendations for products that the patient can purchase. There are a certain number of patients that we see in our pharmacy who think that we are trying to "sell fries with that."

I have a constant job keeping my younger pharmacists motivated and focused on the main issue: optimizing the health of our patients. Sometimes you get several negative patients in a row, so they start to doubt what they are doing. I need to continuously remind my pharmacists that we are the medicine experts and we have a responsibility to our patients to educate them about their health.

We also need to keep reminding ourselves about the costs of not doing our job properly. For example, if a patient leaves our pharmacy with an antibiotic and gets such bad diarrhoea that they have to take a day off work, then that has cost the patient dearly. Or if a patient leaves our pharmacy with their blood pressure and cholesterol medications and falls asleep in front of television every night instead of helping their kids with their homework, that is costly.

Providing education to ensure optimal health is why most pharmacists decided to become pharmacists ... to make a huge difference to the health of every patient. If we don't keep utilizing our best professional skills, then we will soon fall back to become pill counters and Governments rule enforcers. Sadly, in some pharmacies I visit, this is exactly what the pharmacists have become.

How Do I Tell If My Pharmacist Is A Health Expert Or A Pill Counter?

I think the answer to this question is pretty obvious. When you go to collect your prescription, does the pharmacist even bother to discuss your medicines with you? The interaction with the pharmacist is, I believe, the most important part of getting your prescription. When I say this I assume that the technical parts of the job, such as ensuring the prescription is prepared accurately, are done 100% right. Every pharmacist must have 100% accuracy.

But what makes a good pharmacist is the extra mile they go to, to ensure you have the best chance of achieving optimal health. The personal care and attention that they go to. The extra study and knowledge that they acquire so as to pass on to you.

You should ask your pharmacist for their views on complementing your prescription with nutritional supplements. If they are a little vague or dismissive of this, then they probably don't have a good understanding of this area. You could even ask directly what extra courses or qualifications they have that ensures they can easily help you with advice on the safe and effective use of nutritional supplements, including vitamins, minerals and herbs.

For a list of pharmacies with knowledge and expertise in nutrition medicine, see my website

(www.OptimalPrescriptionHealth.co.nz).

Stirring Up A Hornet's Nest

My comments in this chapter may offend some very well meaning pharmacists. It is certainly not my intention to offend anyone. However, when I began my career as a pharmacist, I decided that I would always do what is right rather than just take the easy road. I expect the same dedication to health from my patients too. We all have good days and bad days when our levels of commitment and motivation are either high or low.

But the interesting thing is, once you have your health well under control and have huge reserves of energy and vitality, you find that you can perform at very high levels almost every day.

For example, I have not had a full-blown cold or a flu for about five years now. This is quite an achievement when I am exposed to many sick people almost every day. My success in avoiding the usual winter bugs is related to my diet, lifestyle and supplement regime that keeps my immune system in good shape. I also have some immune boosting nutrients that I keep at work and home, so at the first sign of any sore throat or other symptom, I can give my defence force a big boost. I should mention that your immune system is far more sophisticated and effective than any antibiotic or antiviral medicine ever discovered. But only if you keep your immune system in good running order.

So I am not trying to offend any of my colleagues by mentioning that some pharmacists are better than others. The reaction I hope to get from any pharmacists who read this book, is perhaps to be intrigued to know more, or even better be inspired to learn more about how to ensure their patients can achieve optimal health with every prescription.

Keep Learning

I encourage you all to keep learning about how you can achieve the best health. I will make a commitment to you to continue to share the new information that I discover in my journey to find the real truth about optimal health. I offer this service in the spirit of communing and collaborating, because I firmly believe that by sharing this information with as many people as possible we will all win.

I encourage you to register on my website for my regular health newsletters. I am happy if you also invite your friends and family to also register. The more people that understand the importance of nutrition to health the better. To register for my free newsletter go to www.OptimalPrescriptionHealth.co.nz

13

Change Your Future

Real Life Examples

The information that I have provided in this book has proved life-changing for many of my patients in my pharmacy and in my clinic. Let me give you some examples.

Olivia The 70-Year-Old Golfer

I used to be a keen golfer when I was a teenager. I managed to get my handicap down to 8 when I was 14 years old. But then the lure of a team sport (football) with the camaraderie of my mates (and the potential adoration from girls) saw me shift my focus away from golf. This was back in the late 1970s before inspirational young men like Tiger Woods (before he fell from grace), and the world-beating NZ amateur team (Tautarangi and Campbell) came on the scene. Anyway, I guess I still have a love for the game and when I get more time (probably in about another 40 years or so!) I will dust off my clubs and resurrect my golfing career.

So because of my interest in golf, I often chat about golf with my customers. One of my customers who loves her golf is Olivia. Being in her 70s she has plenty of time for golf. But she mentioned to me the difficulty in moving her fingers in the mornings, and how this was interfering with her golf. So we recommended some fish oils might help. I also suggested that to maintain her energy levels she should also consider coenzyme Q10. Several months later when I saw her I asked how things were progressing. She told me that the previous week on one very hot summers day she had got up early to play golf (no problems with the fingers in the morning), raced home to mow her lawns, then went out in the evening to watch her granddaughter's dance show. Not bad for someone in her 70s!

Doubting Thomas

I was recently wandering through my pharmacy between my appointments with patients in my clinic when I was stopped by Thomas; one of our regular customers.

Thomas called out to me that he had been on antibiotics for some time because of a problem with his waterworks. Now the antibiotics were causing his bowels to play up. He said that he remembers when he picked up his antibiotics in the past, my team had mentioned the importance of taking probiotics to prevent any problems. He admitted that he had been skeptical about our recommendations to complement his prescription and had dismissed our advice.

But after his bowels started playing up he remembered what we had said. So he stopped his antibiotics and his bowels improved. Then he started his antibiotics and things got worse again. I should add here that he did this off his own bat. We wouldn't recommend that he stop his medications without talking to his doctor first.

By now he could feel the problems for himself and he believed. I recommended a course of a quality probiotic for him, which he took.

Thomas is the principal of a local school, so we had a bit of a joke about some people being slower learners than others. I haven't spoken to Thomas since, but my team told me that he purchased a second bottle of probiotics a few weeks later.

Good Healthy Advice

I recommend that you make sure your health advisors, namely your doctor and pharmacist, are skilled in nutrition medicine. Some doctors call themselves "integrated medicine doctors" and this means that they strive to integrate the best of conventional and complementary medicines to ensure you get the best health.

If you are truly committed to embracing both medicines and nutrients then you need a pharmacist and a doctor who can support you on this journey. I strongly believe that you should be embracing both complementary and conventional medicines, since this increases your chances of obtaining true health and vitality, rather than just relieving symptoms.

Change The Game, Eliminate Ill Health

The exciting thing is that more and more doctors and pharmacists are discovering the value of this integrated approach to healthcare. When I first started my learning, there were only a few such health professionals. Tragically, these "trail blazers" had to keep a low profile as they were often persecuted by the medical bodies for being "quacks."

Luckily that is changing now. I received an invitation this week to a conventional medical conference with a sole focus on nutritional medicine. I find it really encouraging that this new science is now becoming more and more mainstream. I truly believe that in another 10 years or so, any health professionals who do not have a full knowledge of nutrition medicine will be left behind like the dinosaurs.

Do You Feel 100%?

Do you take prescription medicines? If so, ask yourself honestly how you feel. Do they make you feel full of energy and vitality? If you answered yes, then fantastic, you are indeed fortunate. If you answered no, then what are you going to do differently to change your health?

Most people will have heard the saying:

"If you always do what you've always done, then you'll always get what you've always got."

In other words, if you want your health to improve, then you need to do something to make it improve.

I have seen dramatic improvements in health with very simple nutrition medicine interventions. I have patients that come back and use the "WOW" word. But to be honest, not everyone gets an instant response. It depends on the patient's initial health, and the type of treatments that we use. I mentioned how the benefits of fish oils can take many months to appear, while coenzyme Q10 can give an instant energy turbo-boost.

Make Great Health One Of Your Long Term Goals

The day-to-day pressures of life often mean that we put our own health and well-being behind more urgent things like the cooking, cleaning, work, and kids activities. So it is important to plan for good health, because if you don't plan for good health it might not happen. Getting an extra half hour in bed in the morning and having to buy junk food for lunch because you have run out of time to make your salmon salad might seem like a good compromise at the time. In fact, you probably won't notice any health problems that day. You may even have a whole week of junk lunches without adverse effects. But look 20 years into the future when you are taking six different medications for your indigestion, irritable bowel, and heart disease. Now you have reduced energy production and it's an even bigger struggle to get out of bed at all. Imagine you being unable to play in the park or on the beach with your grand children. Or not being able to play a full round of golf, or to tend to your vege garden.

In other words, by the time you realize that your health has gone down the drain, you may struggle to get the energy to correct the bad habits of a lifetime. But it's never too late to change.

I guess what I am trying to get you to appreciate is that by setting good health and vitality as one of your long term life goals, this will help you make the right decisions today that will benefit you for the rest of your life.

My Final Words

Actually, these are my final words for this book, not my final final words. I will keep working hard to teach people about how they can optimize their health.

Complementing your prescription medicine is vital to reduce the side effects of medications and help to address the underlying causes of your illness. Our current health system is based on treating populations, so it can often let individual people down. Make sure your doctor and pharmacist are working for you to make sure you get the best outcomes from your prescriptions.

You are the person who is most interested in your health. Don't let uninformed health practitioners rob you of the health and vitality that you can achieve. Remember, the information that I have written in this book is not taught at pharmacy or medical schools. I have taken a great deal of time, energy and money to acquire this knowledge and to put it into a book for you. This information could be life changing. But only if you do something with it.

My plea to you is to **use this information**. Let it make a difference in your life. Plus share it with your friends and loved ones, so they can also discover the truth to great health and vitality.

Remember, knowledge without action is worthless.

Appendix:

24 Good Reasons Why You May Need Nutritional Supplements

1. Poor Digestion

Even when your food intake is good, inefficient digestion can limit your body's uptake of vitamins. Some common causes of inefficient digestion are not chewing well enough and eating too fast. Both of these result in larger than normal food particle size, too large to allow complete action of digestive enzymes. Many people with dentures are unable to chew as efficiently as those with a full set of original teeth.

2. Hot Coffee, Tea And Spices

Habitual drinking of liquids that are too hot, or consuming an excess of irritants such as coffee, tea or pickles and spices can cause inflammation of the digestive linings, resulting in a drop in secretion of digestive fluids and poorer extraction of vitamins and minerals from food.

3. Alcohol

Drinking too much alcohol is known to damage the liver and pancreas, which are vital to digestion and metabolism. It can also damage the lining of the intestinal tract and adversely affect the absorption of nutrients, leading to sub-clinical malnutrition. Regular heavy use of alcohol increases the body's need for the B-group vitamins, particularly thiamine, niacin, pyridoxine, folic acid and vitamins B12, A and C as well as the minerals zinc, magnesium and calcium. Alcohol affects availability, absorption and metabolism of nutrients.

4. Smoking

Smoking tobacco is also an irritant to the digestive tract and increases the metabolic requirements of vitamin C, all else being equal, by at least thirty per cent more than the typical requirements of a non-smoker. Vitamin C, which is normally present in such foods as paw paws, oranges and capsicums, oxidises rapidly once these fruits are cut, juiced, cooked or stored in direct light or near heat. Vitamin C is important for good immune function.

5. Laxatives

Overuse of laxatives can result in poor absorption of vitamins and minerals from food, by hastening the intestinal transit time. Paraffin and other mineral oils increase losses of fat soluble vitamins A, D, E and K. Other laxatives used to excess can cause large losses of minerals such as potassium, sodium and magnesium.

6. Fad Diets

Bizarre diets that miss out on whole groups of foods can be seriously lacking in vitamins. Even the popular low fat diets, if taken to an extreme, can be deficient in vitamins A, D and E. Vegetarian diets, which exclude meat and other animal sources, must be very skilfully planned to avoid vitamin B12 deficiency, which may lead to anaemia.

7. Overcooking

Lengthy cooking or reheating of meat and vegetables can oxidise and destroy heat susceptible vitamins such as the B-group, C and E. Boiling vegetables leaches the water soluble vitamins B-group and C as well as many minerals. Light steaming is preferable. Some vitamins, such as vitamin B6 can be destroyed by irradiation from microwaves.

8. Food Storage

Freezing food containing vitamin E can significantly reduce its levels once defrosted. Foods containing vitamin E exposed to heat and air can turn rancid. Many common sources of vitamin E, such as bread and oils are nowadays highly processed, so that the vitamin E content is significantly reduced or missing totally, which increases storage life but can lower nutrient levels. Vitamin E is an antioxidant which defensively inhibits oxidative damage to all tissues. Other vitamin losses from food preserving can include vitamin B1 and C.

9. Convenience Foods

A diet overly dependent on highly refined carbohydrates, such as sugar, white flour and white rice places greater demand on additional sources of B-group vitamins to process these carbohydrates. An unbalanced diet contributes to such conditions as irritability, lethargy and sleep disorders.

10. Antibiotics

Some antibiotics although valuable in fighting infection, also kill off friendly bacteria in the gut, which would normally be producing B-group vitamins to be absorbed through the intestinal walls. Such deficiencies can result in a variety of nervous conditions, therefore it may be advisable to supplement with B-group vitamins when on a lengthy course of broad-spectrum antibiotics, and/or use pure lactobacillus powders.

11. Food Allergies

The omission of whole food groups from the diet, as in the case of individuals allergic to gluten or lactose, can mean the loss of significant dietary sources of nutrients such as thiamine, riboflavin or calcium.

12. Crop Nutrient Losses

Some agricultural soils are deficient in trace elements. Decades of intensive agriculture can overwork and deplete soils, unless all the soil nutrients, including trace elements, are regularly replaced. In one US Government survey, levels of essential minerals in crops were found to have declined by up to 68 per cent over a four year period in the 1970's.

13. Accidents And Illnesses

Burns lead to a loss of protein and essential trace nutrients such as vitamins and minerals. Surgery increases the need for zinc, vitamin E and other nutrients involved in the cellular repair mechanism. The repair of broken bones will be retarded by an inadequate supply of calcium and vitamin C and conversely enhanced by a full dietary supply. The challenge of infection places high demand on the nutritional resources of zinc, magnesium and vitamins B5, B6 and zinc.

14. Stress

Chemical, physical and emotional stresses can increase the body's requirements for vitamins B2, B5, B6 and C. Air pollution increases the requirements for vitamin E.

15. P.M.T.

Research has demonstrated that up to 60 per cent of women

suffering from symptoms of premenstrual tension, such as head-aches, irritability, bloatedness, breast tenderness, lethargy and depression can benefit from supplementation with B6.

16. Teenagers

Rapid growth spurts such as in the teenage years, particularly in girls, place high demands on nutritional resources to underwrite the accelerated physical, bio-chemical and emotional develop-ment in this age group. Data from the USA Ten State Nutri-tion Survey in 1968-1970, covering a total of 24,000 families and 86,000 individuals, showed that between 30-50 per cent of adolescents aged 12 to 16 had dietary intakes below two-thirds of the recommended daily averages for vitamin A, C, calcium and iron.

17. Pregnant Women

Pregnancy creates higher than average demands for nutrients, to ensure healthy growth of the baby and comfortable confinement for the mother. Nutrients which typically require increase dur-ing pregnancy are the B-group, especially B1, B2, B3, B6, folic acid and B12, A, D, E and the minerals calcium, iron, magne-sium, zinc, and phosphorous. The Ten State Nutrition Survey in the USA in 1968-70 showed that as many as 80 per cent of the pregnant women surveyed had dietary intakes below two thirds of recommended daily allowances. Professional assessment of nutrient requirements during pregnancy should be sought.

18. Oral Contraceptives

Oral contraceptives can decrease absorption of folic acid and increase the need for vitamin B6, and possibly vitamin C, zinc and riboflavin. Approximately 22 per cent of Australian women aged 15-44 are believed to be on "the pill" at any one time.

19. Light Eaters

Some people eat very sparingly, even without weight reduction goals. US dietary surveys have shown that an average woman maintains her weight on 7560 kilojoules per day, at which level her diet is likely to be low in thiamine, calcium and iron.

20. The Elderly

The aged have been shown to have a low intake of vitamins and minerals, particularly iron, calcium and zinc. Folic acid deficiency is often found in conjunction with vitamin C deficiency. Fibre intake is often low. Riboflavine (B2) and pyridoxine (B6) deficiencies have also been observed. Possible causes include impaired sense of taste and smell, reduced secretion of digestive enzymes, chronic disease and maybe, physical impairment.

21. Lack Of Sunlight

Invalids, shiftworkers and people whose exposure to sunlight may be minimal can suffer from insufficient amounts of vitamin D, which is required for calcium metabolism, without which rickets and osteoporosis (bone thinning) has been observed.

Ultraviolet light is the stimulus to vitamin D formation in skin. It is blocked by cloud, fog, smog, ordinary window glass, curtains and clothing. The maximum recommended daily supplemental intake of vitamin D is 100 IU.

22. Bio-Individuality

Wide fluctuations in individual nutrient requirements from the official recommended average vitamin and mineral intakes are common, particularly for those in high physical demand vocations, such as athletes and manual labour, taking into account body weight and physical type. Protein intake influences the need for vitamin B6 and vitamin B1 is linked to kilojoules intake.

23. Low Body Reserves

Although the body is able to store reserves of certain vitamins such as A and E, Canadian autopsy data has shown that up to thirty per cent of the population have reserves of vitamin A so low as to be judged "at risk." Vitamin A is important to healthy skin and mucous membranes (including sinus and lungs) and eyesight.

24. Athletes

Athletes consume large amounts of food and experience considerable stress. These factors affect their needs for B-group vitamins, vitamin C and iron in particular. Tests on Australian Olympic athletes and A-grade football players, for example, have shown wide-ranging vitamin deficiencies.

Special Bonus Offer
Nutricheck Health Analysis
For you and a loved one
Plus a 20 minute personal health consultation
(either face-to-face or via Skype or Phone)

(Valued at $280)

A Nutricheck Health Analysis is an important step in your journey to wellness.

What the Nutricheck Health Analysis will do for you:
- You will discover how likely it is that your health condition is actually caused by a deficiency of one or more nutrients.
- You will discover what nutrients your body is crying out for.
- Your Nutricheck report will reveal if your prescription drugs have caused low levels of essential nutrients.
- You will receive your own personalized plan to assist you to achieve Optimal Health.

As a bonus gift for investing in this book, you can claim your FREE GIFT of a Nutricheck Health Analysis.

To claim your Nutricheck Health Analysis please register at:
www.OptimalPrescriptionHealth.co.nz

This offer is open to all acquirers of Optimal Prescription Health, The Real Truth About Balancing Your Prescription With Complementary Medicines, How A Good Pharmacist Can Save Your Life, by Martin Harris. Original proof of purchase is required. This offer is limited to the Nutricheck Health Analysis and a 20 minute consultation only (in person, or remotely by Phone or Skype), and your appointment will be subject to availability of appointments. The appointments must be completed by **1 December 2012.** The value of this Nutricheck Health Analysis for you and a loved one is $280 as of April 2011. While book purchasers will be responsible for the travel, meals, accommodation and other expenses, the Nutricheck Health Analysis is complimentary. In undertaking a Nutricheck Health Analysis you are under no obligation whatsoever to Martin Harris, his pharmacy or his clinic.